D1686104

THE CERTIFICATION AND RECERTIFICATION OF DOCTORS: ISSUES IN THE ASSESSMENT OF CLINICAL COMPETENCE

THE CERTIFICATION AND RECERTIFICATION OF DOCTORS: ISSUES IN THE ASSESSMENT OF CLINICAL COMPETENCE

Edited by

DAVID NEWBLE
Associate Professor, Department of Medicine, University of Adelaide, South Australia, Australia

BRIAN JOLLY
Senior Lecturer, Joint Academic Unit of Medical and Dental Education, St Bartholomew's and the London Hospital's Medical Colleges, London, UK

RICHARD WAKEFORD
Educational Advisor, School of Clinical Medicine, Cambridge University, Cambridge, UK

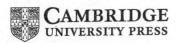
CAMBRIDGE
UNIVERSITY PRESS

Published by the Press Syndicate of the University of Cambridge
The Pitt Building, Trumpington Street, Cambridge CB2 1RP
40 West 20th Street, New York, NY 10011–4211, USA
10 Stamford Road, Oakleigh, Melbourne 3166, Australia

First published 1994

Printed in Great Britain at the University Press, Cambridge

A catalogue record for this book is available from the British Library

Library of Congress cataloguing in publication data

The certification and recertification of doctors: issues in the assessment of clinical
competence/edited by David Newble, Brian Jolly, Richard Wakeford.
   p. cm.
Includes index
ISBN 0-521-43187-5 (hardback)
1. Physicians–Certification–Congresses. I. Newble, David.
II. Jolly, Brian. III. Wakeford, R. E. (Richard E.)
[DNLM: 1. Certification–congresses. 2. Clinical Competence–congresses.
W 21 C418 1993]
RA396.A1C47   1993
362. 1'72–dc20   92-48562 CIP

ISBN 0 521 43187 5 hardback

Contents

Contributors

Associate Professor Raja Bandaranayake
School of Medical Education, University of NSW, PO Box 1, Kensington, NSW 2033, Australia

Dr Ian Bowmer
Health Sciences Centre, Memorial University, St John's, Newfoundland, Canada A1B 3V6

Dr Donald Cameron
Princess Alexandra Hospital, Ipswich Road, Woolloongabba, Brisbane, Qld 4102, Australia

Dr Susan Case
National Board of Medical Examiners, 3930 Chestnut Street, Philadelphia, PA 19104, USA

Dr Dale Dauphinee
Center for Medical Education, Lady Meredith House, 1110 Pine Avenue West, Montreal, QUE, Canada H3A 1A3

Dr Wayne Davis
G1111 Towsley Center, University of Michigan Medical School, Ann Arbor, MI 48109–0201, USA

Dr Beth Dawson-Saunders
Division of Informatics, Biostatistics and Research, Southern Illinois University, School of Medicine, Springfield, IL 62794, USA

Dr Jean-Pierre des Groseilliers
Royal College of Physicians and Surgeons of Canada, 74 Stanley Street, Ottawa, ONT, Canada K1M 1P4

Dr Jacques des Marchais
Université de Sherbrooke, Faculty of Medicine, 3001 12e Avenue N, Sherbrooke, QUE, Canada J1H 5N4

Dr Brendan Dooley
141 Grey Street, East Melbourne, Victoria 3002, Australia

Dr Wesley Fabb
Royal Australian College of General Practitioners, 70 Jolimont Street, East Melbourne, Victoria 3002, Australia

Dr Elizabeth Farmer
Family Medicine Programme, Royal Australian College of General Practitioners, 15 Gover Street, North Adelaide, SA 5006, Australia

Dr Grahame Feletti
Ke Ola O Hawaii, Inc, Leahl Hospital, 3675 Kilavea Avenue, Honolulu, HA 96816, USA

Dr John Foulkes
University of Cambridge Local Examinations Syndicate, 1 Hills Road, Cambridge CB1 2EU, UK

Dr Roger Gabb
Royal Australian College of Obstetricians and Gynaecologists, 254 Albert Street, East Melbourne, Victoria 3002, Australia

Professor Richard Hays
Department of General Practice and Rural Health, North Queensland Clinical School, Townsville, QLD 4810, Australia

Dr Gareth Holsgrove
Joint Academic Unit of Medical and Dental Education, St Bartholomew's and the London Hospital's Medical Colleges, Charterhouse Square, London EC1M 6BQ, UK

Mr Brian Jolly
Joint Academic Unit of Medical and Dental Education, St Bartholomew's and the London Hospital's Medical Colleges, Charterhouse Square, London EC1M 6BQ, UK

Dr Donald Langsley
American Board of Medical Specialties, 1 Rotary Center, No. 805, Evanston, IL 60201, USA

Ms Morag MacDonald
8 St Fillans Terrace, Edinburgh EH10 5NH, Scotland

Dr Pauline McAvoy
Department of General Practice, University of Auckland, Private Bag, Auckland, New Zealand

Dr Barrie McCann
Faculty of Anaesthetists, Royal Australasian College of Surgeons, c/o PO Box 239, Spring Hill, Qld 4004, Australia

Dr Colin McRae
Milford Chambers, 249 Papanui Road, Christchurch, 1, New Zealand

Dr Helen Mulholland
Centre for Medical Education, Ninewells Hospital and Medical School, Dundee DD1 9SY, Scotland

Associate Professor David Newble
University of Adelaide, Department of Medicine, Queen Elizabeth Hospital, Woodville, SA 5011, Australia

Dr John Norcini
American Board of Internal Medicine, 3624 Market Street, Philadelphia, PA 19104, USA

Dr Gordon Page
Division of Educational Support and Development, Office of the Coordinator of Health Sciences, 2194 Health Sciences Mall, Vancouver, BC, Canada V6T 1Z6

Dr Garry Phillips
Department of Anaesthesia and Intensive Care, Flinders Medical Centre, Bedford Park, SA 5042, Australia

Dr Peter Procopis
Australian College of Paediatrics, Royal Alexandra Hospital for Children, Camperdown, NSW 2050, Australia

Dr Arthur Rothman
Department of Medicine, University of Toronto, 100 College Street, #526, Toronto, ONT, Canada M5G 1L5

Professor Nicholas Saunders
Flinders University of South Australia, Faculty of Medicine, Bedford Park, SA 5042, Australia

Professor Lesley Southgate
Department of General Practice, St Bartholomew's and the London Hospital's Medical Colleges, Charterhouse Square, London EC1M 6BQ, UK

Dr David Swanson
National Board of Medical Examiners, 3938 Chestnut Street, Philadelphia, PA 19104, USA

Dr Alex Thomson
Department of General Practice, School of Medicine, University of Auckland, Auckland, New Zealand

Dr Cees van der Vleuten
Educational Research and Development, Faculty of Medicine, Rijksuniversiteit Limburg, 6200 Maastricht, The Netherlands

Mr Richard Wakeford
School of Clinical Medicine, Cambridge University, Addenbrooke's Hospital, Cambridge CB2 2SP, UK

Dr Stephen Wealthall
School of Medicine, University of Auckland, Private Bag, Auckland, New Zealand

Dr Gregory Whelan
Department of Community Medicine, St Vincent's Hospital, Fitzroy, Victoria 3065, Australia

Preface

The certification and recertification of the clinical competence of doctors are issues which have been of growing concern in recent years. In 1984, a highly selected international group of researchers and practising clinicians, with a common interest in clinical assessment, met in Cambridge (UK) to undertake a 'state of the art review' and to prepare a research agenda of the major issues in the evaluation of clinical competence. The success of this 'think tank' led to further Cambridge Conferences on Medical Education which dealt with other important educational topics such as selection and curriculum development. However, the major focus remained on assessment. The Fourth Conference in 1989 provided a follow-up to the inaugural meeting.

The aim of the Fifth Conference, held in Adelaide, Australia, in 1991, was somewhat different. The main purpose was to discuss the integration and implementation of the recent advances in assessment methodology into the practices of universities, colleges and specialty boards. Those invited to attend formed a balance of clinicians, psychometricians, educational researchers and policy makers from universities and national certification and licensing organizations from Australasia, North America, the United Kingdom and the Netherlands. The impact on those policy makers attending the Conference has been profound, with much activity being generated, particularly within the Royal Colleges.

This publication is a major component of a strategy to extend the outcome of the Conference beyond those fortunate enough to attend. It is hoped that it will stimulate discussion and assist in the introduction of long-overdue changes to assessment practices in both the undergraduate and postgraduate arenas.

The book is divided into four parts. The first is an introductory part which looks broadly at the current issues in certification and recertification. The second part contains a series of articles, initially prepared as background papers for the Conference. They provide an international perspective on current and projected practice in certification and recertification.

The third part consists of chapters which relate to the initial certification of competence. It commences with a chapter, previously published as an occasional paper from the Fourth Cambridge Conference, which describes guidelines for the development of procedures for the assessment of clinical competence. These guidelines provide a starting point for many of the chapters to follow. This chapter is followed by others generated from the Conference on aspects of certification. The fourth part contains the chapters which relate to ensuring the competence of doctors through recertification. Each chapter in these two parts represents the output of a small group of participants who worked for three days during the Conference and subsequently by correspondence. While the organizers of the Conference selected the topics to cover a range of relevant issues there is, inevitably, a variability in the depth and breadth of coverage in the papers. There is also a degree of overlap. Nevertheless a policy decision was made by the editors and the Conference not overly to influence the individuality of, and intellectual input into, each chapter.

The book concludes with a brief discussion of the implications for action and future research.

The authors wish to acknowledge the financial support of the following organizations which made it possible to conduct the Fifth Cambridge Conference and produce this book:
Australian Medical Council
British Council
Faculty of Anaesthetists, Royal Australasian College of Surgeons
Royal Australasian College of Physicians
Royal Australasian College of Surgeons
Royal Australian College of General Practitioners
Royal Australian College of Obstetricians and Gynaecologists
University of Adelaide, Faculty of Medicine
University of Adelaide Foundation

The editors and contributors to this book owe a considerable intellectual debt to the First Cambridge Conference, in particular to the participants who generated so much of the early goodwill and research effort. They include Philip Bashook, Georges Bordage, Colin Coles, Lynn Curry, Charles Friedman, J.-J. Guilbert, Dick Martenson, Geoff Norman, Gordon Page, David Pendleton, Clive Quick, Ed Sellers, Betsy

Stalenhoef, Paula Stillman, Dave Swanson, Xenia Tonesk, Ragnar Tunell and Iain Wilkinson.

The authors also thank Kathryn Heaton and all the other staff at the conference venue, Leonard's Mill in Second Valley, South Australia.

Garry Raymond provided an invaluable contribution by shouldering much of the organizational burden of the conference. He has also been responsible for coordinating the secretarial work involved in producing the typescript for this book, a task in which he was ably assisted by Ermioni Mourtzios and Tracy Chinner.

D. N.
B. J.
R. W.

Part A

Introduction

1

Background to the conference and issues in certification and recertification

DAVID NEWBLE, BRIAN JOLLY and
RICHARD WAKEFORD

The last two decades have seen major developments in the assessment
of clinical competence. This has been evident in the amount of research
and written output in this area of medical education and in the number
of major international conferences which have focused on this topic.
Published examples include: the 'Ottawa' Conferences, a series of
international conferences on the teaching and assessment of clinical
competence (1985, 1987, 1989, 1990, 1992); the First (1984) and Fourth
(1989) Cambridge Conferences on Medical Education; and the more
established annual conferences of organizations such as the Association
for Medical Education in Europe (1980). However, this unprecedented
interest, at best, has led to a patchy introduction of change in the
approaches used by organizations and institutions which have the responsibility for implementing examinations and other forms of assessment relating to certification and recertification. Despite the efforts of
educational researchers to provide the evidence often demanded by
medical academics and leaders of the profession, valuable data have all
too often remained unknown, unavailable or unaccepted. Feeling that
this was a major issue which no longer could be ignored, the organizers
of the Cambridge Conferences set out to arrange a meeting of minds
between educational researchers, who had made substantial contributions to the development of new approaches to the assessment of
clinical competence, and those responsible within universities, boards
and colleges for administering certification examinations and recertification procedures. The aim was to identify and debate the issues and then
to put forward practical suggestions for immediate action and future
research.

3

International perspectives

Something that becomes immediately apparent when one looks at the issues of assessment of competence from an international perspective is the marked variability between countries in both policies and procedures despite broadly similar goals. Much of what occurs in practice seems to be determined more by traditionally and historically based practices than by the rational use of approaches and methods chosen for their proven value. Similar reasons seem to have determined the nature and function of the official bodies with responsibility for certification. For example, Chapter 2 reviews the certification procedures which hold sway in the United Kingdom (UK) and Australasia where national medical councils control both undergraduate training and primary certification, but indirectly through a process of accrediting the medical school curriculum. The medical school itself is responsible for assessment and standard setting. In North America (see Chapter 3) the medical schools have less authority in this regard, with national examinations playing a major role in certification. The former approach has potential advantages in terms of flexibility but disadvantages in terms of the psychometric quality of the locally produced assessment procedures. There is no doubt that central examination-producing organizations, such as the American National Board of Medical Examiners, have set standards of technical quality which are hard to match by institutions with limited resources and educational expertise.

In the area of specialty certification there is more common ground, yet still more significant differences. Again, it is interesting to contrast the situation in the UK and Australasia with that in North America. In the former, responsibility lies with the nationally based Colleges, which are both the certifying body and the professional organization for the specialty. In the latter, assessment is undertaken by national boards, for which this is their sole responsibility.

These differences reflect not only historical precedents but also cultural, political and social differences, both past and present. Medical educators and measurement specialists may agree on desirable approaches to assessment but these may not be acceptable in a particular country or institution for a variety of reasons. Good examples of this variation are seen in the area of recertification (see Chapters 4, 5, 12 and 16).

The lack of common procedures for certification causes considerable difficulties in the acceptance of qualifications in different countries and sometimes even between states or provinces of one country. This is currently causing particular problems for countries accepting refugee or immigrant doctors whose basic qualifications are unacceptable to licensing bodies. This usually leads to the establishment of special competency-based examinations which inevitably become a matter of controversy with accusations of standards being set too high or being racially biased. When countries move towards political union, as is occurring currently in Europe, particular problems are posed when educational systems, certifying practices and assessment standards are different.

The overall picture is one where entry requirements into the profession (primary certification) and subsequently into a specialty (secondary certification) are strong and rigorous. The purpose of the assessment task is usually clear. The same cannot be said of recertification, where policies and procedures are less well developed. There is an ambivalence about the purpose of recertification with the profession being concerned more with personal development and maintenance of standards, while the government and community, from whom the stimulus for recertification may be arising, are concerned more about deregistering those who are incompetent – often referred to as 'identifying the bad apples'. The threads of this issue are pulled together in Chapters 4 and 5.

The assessment methods used in most countries for certification purposes have a degree of commonality which has become more evident in recent years. New methods, particularly those directed at clinical performance, are being actively introduced into both national and institution-based assessments. Good examples of this include the widespread use of objective structured clinical examinations and the increasing use of standardized patients (i.e. people trained to simulate a range of clinical features, who, in addition, may be trained to assess the performance of the student). This rapid transfer of methods, which were often developed in one or two countries, reflects the common perceived objectives for primary and secondary certification. Once again this can be contrasted with recertification where there are major differences between countries in approach and methods. In the UK, Australasia and, rather surprisingly, Canada, the approach to recertification is predominantly through maintenance of competence, using participation in continuing medical education and other professional development activities as the criteria of achievement (see Chapter 5). In America, the trend is strongly in the direction of recertification by demonstration of competence based on formal examinations and audit of practice and patient outcomes (see Chapter 4).

Issues for certification

Defining content and determining methods

An issue of prime importance is the need to define quite explicitly what is expected of the candidate. For a competency examination the content ought to be related primarily to the required on-the-job performance, the clinical milieu into which the candidate is to move, whether this be an internship, residency or specialty practice. This definition must be broadly based to include value laden aspects as well as strictly medical tasks. A model for developing a competence examination was one outcome of the Fourth Cambridge Conference (Chapter 6) and was used as a starting point for further discussion at this conference (Chapter 7). The key points of this model are: that the content should be defined in terms of real-life presenting problems; that for each problem the specific knowledge, tasks and actions required to deal with each problem must be specified at the expected level of performance (intern, specialist); and that a blueprint be produced to provide a concrete framework for sampling and method selection. This general approach was supported and further developed as a key element in any strategy to upgrade current assessment procedures.

It could be said that the range of methods is now so comprehensive that few issues remain in test development. It is certainly true that there is a wealth of current and well referenced information. However, some aspects of competency testing are still poorly served by present test technology. This applies particularly to that of clinical problem-solving. Nevertheless, the major need is to discard procedures which incorporate methods with proven limitations of reliability and validity and to replace them with those having a better assessment profile.

Other issues of concern, which are discussed in Chapter 8, include the recognition of the impact of test methods and the content of assessments on student learning and the problem of 'content specificity'. The latter is now a recognized limitation of all methods used to assess competence – the poor generalizability of performance across items or tasks. The universal implication of this is that most tests of competence have to be much longer and more complex than those commonly in use. This unpopular fact has in itself triggered a search for more efficient testing strategies.

Standard setting

The setting of standards is an aspect of competence testing that often receives scant attention. As a result, practices are frequently primitive, unprofessional and more arbitrary than they ought to be. The commonly used relative (norm-referenced) standards are increasingly being challenged and a strong trend is evident towards absolute (criterion-referenced; competency-based) standards. There is a growing demand from without for more scrutiny of standards (even legal challenges) and for evidence of fairness and lack of bias. A critical look at current practices often reveals many deficiencies. Unfortunately, the methodology for absolute standard setting is underdeveloped and little work has been done outside that on conventional written tests of knowledge. These issues are pursued in Chapter 9.

Combining components

It is a common procedure to combine examination components to produce a final score. The hazards and pitfalls of doing so are seldom given a passing thought, except by professional examining bodies. Thus, Chapter 10 may be a revelation to many of those responsible for running multi-component examinations. The increasing use of batteries of test methods in competence testing makes it essential to look more carefully at this issue. Failure to adopt appropriate procedures will lead to unintended outcomes which may distort the whole purpose of the assessment.

In-training evaluation

Assessment of competence for certification purposes has been heavily weighted in favour of some form of final examination. However, new perspectives on measuring competence, which focus more on the content and context, inevitably lead one to reappraise the pre-eminent role of a single, end-of-course evaluation. Some important components of competence simply cannot be measured in an examination, requiring as they do direct observation of performance in the actual clinical setting. Once this is accepted as an essential component of the assessment procedure the known weaknesses of direct assessment have to be faced. The issue becomes one of applying the same rigour to the development of standardization in this setting as has occurred for the clinical examination (e.g. replacing traditional clinical vivas with structured clinical examinations). Chapter 11 proposes several models of assessment with a variable role for in-training assessment.

Issues for recertification

While many of the issues for recertification are common to those of certification, others are unique or pose considerably greater problems. The interplay between political and educational factors is much more evident, with the former often predominating. Much of what is current is in a state of flux, there being little or no tradition of recertification from which to evolve. Direct transfer of experience from certification is often not appropriate.

Policy considerations

Despite being heavily politicized, continuing medical education and recertification are among the most under-developed, under-resourced and under-researched areas of medical education. This means that major decisions on policy and implementation are being made on the basis of inadequate data and experience. The relationship between the certifying, and hence recertifying, bodies, and those who hold the power over licensure has produced widely differing approaches between countries and even between different specialty groups within one country. Looking at it from the point-of-view of the medical profession, a policy which gives priority to the maintenance of competence for the whole profession is seen as the most desirable aim. An external agency (government, licensing authority, community) may be happy to accept this as a general approach. However, it would be surprising if they did not also demand an assurance that incompetent practitioners would be identified reliably and their certification withdrawn if they failed to achieve a defined minimum standard. In some communities this may be the main pressure for recertification and the demand for a rigorous objective assessment may force the profession into a procedure based on formal testing. These issues and the implications they have for implementation are discussed in Chapter 12.

Defining content and determining methods

In principle, the same approach advocated for certification can be applied to recertification. Indeed, the imperative for such an approach is even more compelling. An assessment of the competence of a clinician must be based on the job performed in practice if it is to be valid – and an invalid test should never be countenanced. However, the complexity of this task goes well beyond that required for primary and secondary certification, where common hurdles are relatively easy to define. This is an area where considerable creativity will be required and Chapter 13 develops a four-level model reflecting the need to include in the assessment: a core of characteristics common to all doctors; a representation of the primary and secondary levels of specialization of the individual practitioner; and a measure of performance in actual practice.

The logic of such an approach is hard to fault but it has enormous implications for the choice of methods of assessment. Chapter 14 looks at the choice of methods by using the general practitioner, the specialist in private practice and the specialist based in a teaching hospital as exemplars for possible certification procedures.

Standard setting

The need to assess individuals in recertification provides enormous difficulties and challenges for standard setting if recertification by examination is to proceed. Clarification of the purpose of the recertification process and the basis on which unsatisfactory performance is to be judged will be critical. The decisions that are to be made when someone is thought to be unsatisfactory have vital consequences for the practitioner concerned. The issue of standard setting does not only apply to procedures based on examinations but also to procedures based on satisfactory participation in maintenance of competence programmes. In the latter, standards must be set for the quality of the components of the programme and for levels of active participation. Chapter 15 contains a detailed discussion of these matters with illustrative examples.

Implementation

Implementing a recertification procedure may be far more complex and difficult than might be anticipated. Chapter 16 focuses on a real example of a college which introduced compulsory recertification as part of its charter. Emphasis is placed on the widespread involvement of the members, the need for both internal and external public relations; the appointment and training of staff, and evaluation. Resources, administrative arrangements and legally defensible processes have to be clearly defined.

Issues for action and research

There is no doubt that the assessment of clinical competence is one of the topics in medical education which has benefited from a period of sustained and fruitful research. Enough 'hard evidence' has been produced to convince the most sceptical that there is a need for change in our certification and recertification procedures.

In the concluding chapter an attempt is made to identify areas not only where further research is required, but also where opportunities exist for more immediate action. General trends are emerging which will influence these developments. Examples include the need to base assessments in more realistic settings but in ways which are psychometrically respectable. Blueprints will be used more extensively to improve content validity and more comprehensive but efficient procedures will emerge to deal with the problem of content specificity.

In the field of recertification, major debates continue on several issues. One which requires early resolution is the need to decide the relative values to be given to evaluating the core or generic skills of medical practice and to the knowledge and skills which are context and specialty specific.

Recent psychological research on clinical problem-solving has highlighted the critical importance of developing innovative methods of testing problem-solving, one of the components of competence where current methodology is largely discredited.

Standard setting is also emerging as an area where present procedures are weak. This results partly from inadequate statistical practices and partly from the lack of suitable methods of setting standards for many of the new approaches to clinical performance-based assessments.

Part B

International background and perspectives

2

Primary certification in the UK and Australasia

DAVID NEWBLE and RICHARD WAKEFORD

To understand the process of certification and registration to practise medicine in the UK and Australasia it is helpful to take a historical perspective.

The British system of medical education was transported to Australia and New Zealand in colonial days and to this day close similarities exist. In the early nineteenth century, there were increasing concerns in the UK about the unregulated system of medical practice (Rhodes, 1985). Until 1858, 19 separate licensing bodies awarded medical titles, using widely varying tests. The qualifications mostly had local value only. This lack of system, the inadequate tests for many of the qualifications and the large number of wholly uncertified practitioners made it impossible for the public to distinguish qualified from unqualified persons (W. K. Pyke Lees (1958) quoted by Anon. (1977)).

British Government intervention led to the passage of the Medical Act of 1858 which established the General Medical Council (GMC). Effectively, it regulated entry to the profession by establishing a Medical Register in which only those with approved qualifications were to be included.

In order to do this, the GMC had to determine what the doctor needed to know and what training was necessary. Therefore, it set guidelines for the curriculum of the medical schools, irrespective of whether they were university-based or hospital-based (then the common pattern in London). In addition to this, the GMC was given the right to visit and to approve (or to disapprove of) the curriculum of institutions where medical education was undertaken and to inspect their examinations.

Thus a process has developed whereby standards and external supervision are imposed for all aspects of education, not just examination procedures. This same process is in operation today in the UK and almost identical ones are to be seen in Australia and New Zealand. It is only recently that the Australian Medical Council (AMC) has been established to take over the role of the GMC. It is expected that in the near future the Medical Council of New Zealand will also obtain statutory responsibility for overviewing medical education.

Registration

Registration (licensure) in the UK is still a GMC function and is available only to those who have graduated from an approved institution.

In Australia, registration is the function of State (or Territory) Medical Boards. Their role is simply to make decisions about the qualifications of applicants which they may or may not accredit. In the past there have been varying requirements, which have caused some difficulties. Agreement on standard registration requirements among all Boards will be in place shortly. Those whose credentials are not acceptable have to pass an examination, now conducted by the AMC. This is a matter of considerable controversy with large numbers of foreign medical graduates seeking the right to practise. A similar registration situation obtains in New Zealand, with the responsible body being its Medical Council.

Recommendations on basic medical education

The Education Committee of the GMC is by statute an independent body. It has a defined membership, about half of whom are representatives of either the medical schools (e.g. deans) or the Royal Colleges. It is this body which is effectively responsible for accrediting medical schools and approving their examinations.

To guide medical schools, the Education Committee periodically publishes *Recommendations on Basic Medical Education* (which includes the preregistration or intern year over which it also has regulatory powers) (GMCEC, 1980). Although these recommendations include guidelines for assessments and examinations, they are neither prescriptive nor required absolutely. However, they indicate the general directions in which the Education Committee thinks procedures should go and even recommend the range of methods which might be used. For instance, the *Recommendations* (1980, p. 25) state that 'The Council believes that special weight should be given to the student's record throughout the course, and recommends that a system of continuous or progressive assessment should be established and maintained for this purpose'. Even so, it is recognized that the particular arrangement must depend to a large extent on the teaching methods and programmes in each individual medical school.

The document makes general recommendations about the necessity for qualifying examinations, which may either be a final examination or may be conducted in stages and in conjunction with progressive assessment. It advises multiple formats of written tests of knowledge and states that an examination in clinical skills is an indispensable part of the qualifying examination. In such examinations the involvement of two assessors is advised to reduce bias.

While not itself conducting national assessments, the GMC asks that external examiners take part in the examination of students. This may include monitoring written examinations but always implies involvement in clinical and other viva voce examinations. Their potential influence on pass–fail decision-making is seen as important in all institutions. Such examiners are also expected by the medical school to provide feedback on their impressions of the form of assessment and standard of the students.

The GMC's latest *Review of Undergraduate Medical Education* is under consideration by the Deans of medical schools (GMCEC, 1991). The main concern appears to be radical change to the curriculum advocating a 'core plus options' approach. Limited reference only is made to assessment issues.

In Australia, a very similar situation obtains. However, the AMC is now taking a more forceful approach than does its UK counterpart. In recent years, the latter has never failed to approve medical schools' courses and examinations (though frequently with modest comment and criticism). The AMC has embarked upon a programme of accreditation visits and on occasions has awarded limited accreditation only. This had enormous impact on these institutions and on other institutions awaiting accreditation. Currently it is still using the GMC *Recommendations* but is in the process of preparing its own.

The Medical Council of New Zealand recently commissioned a review of undergraduate medical education (Renwick *et al.*, 1988). Changes to the Medical Practitioners Act were recommended which would give the Council statutory responsibility for supervising medical education. It was also recommended that the Education Committee should produce its own recommendations on curricula and should undertake regular accreditation reviews. Joint procedures with the AMC were envisaged.

Current situation

The system of external regulation of the curriculum by a body such as the GMC or AMC means that the medical schools have a large degree of autonomy with regard to their assessment and certification procedures. To all intents and purposes the award of the medical degree is also a certificate of competence to practise in the preregistration year. This has advantages and limitations.

The advantages relate to the flexibility that the arrangement allows, with opportunities to assess a wider range of skills in a variety of settings than can be achieved in a nationally based examination. This is particularly evident with clinical assessment, which is highly valued by the institutions. The flexibility has also allowed the introduction of new methods of assessment, such as the objective structured clinical examination (OSCE), without the need for the massive resources which would be required to introduce this into a national assessment scheme.

The limitations relate largely to the fact that the format of the examinations owes more to historically based tradition and rites of passage than to psychometric considerations. This is particularly so with regard to clinical assessment, with medical schools and postgraduate specialist colleges continuing to use the 'traditional clinical oral examination', unfazed by a wealth of evidence concerning its unreliability (Hubbard *et al.*, 1965; Hubbard, 1971). This may be due partly to the high face validity of the approach but may also be attributable to the fact that there have been few pressures to change. Indeed, many would say that this characterizes assessment in UK medical education. Little attention is given to the statistical procedures from which the technical limitations of this format would become evident (Stokes, 1974).

Medical schools in the UK and Australasia rarely employ educational specialists who would bring psychometric matters to the attention of Boards of Examiners. As a result there is a paucity of published data on the reliability and validity of traditional medical school examinations, though such information is becoming available for some of the more innovative approaches (Newble & Swanson, 1988).

Generally speaking, medical schools are bemused and resentful when the validity and reliability of their procedures are challenged. Nevertheless, it is possible to detect a slight breeze of change. In a *Lancet* editorial (Anon, 1991) it has been suggested that one of the implications of the GMC proposals for undergraduate medical education will be a move towards a national assessment procedure.

In Australia, the Department of Employment, Education and Training (DEET) is promoting national standards for 'competency-based skills assessment' in the professions (Heywood *et al.*, 1992). Controversy surrounding the AMC's examinations for foreign medical graduates has attracted the attention of the DEET and the debate now involves the university medical schools and the Colleges. A national workshop on this issue was arranged by the AMC to coincide with the Fifth Cambridge Conference and the presence in Australia of its experts.

Whilst requiring critical review, assessment procedures in the UK and Australasia have some strengths. Our view is that the examination and assessment procedures can be made more reliable and comparable and appropriate standards between schools can be assured. The GMC and the AMC could do much to enhance this process by defining the expected standards for assessment procedures. This possibility was also suggested by Lazarus *et al.* (1976) following a survey of the structure, character and results of the final examinations held in the UK. Failure to achieve standardization will create pressures for some form of national assessment.

References

Anon. (1977). *Basic Medical Education in the British Isles*. Report of the GMC Survey, London: Nuffield Provincial Hospitals Trust.

Anon. (1991). Pulling British medical education into the twentieth century. [Editorial.] *Lancet*, **337**, 1448–9.

GMCEC (General Medical Council Education Committee) (1980). *Recommendations on Basic Medical Education*. London: General Medical Council.

GMCEC (General Medical Council Education Committee) (1991). *Review of Undergraduate Medical Education*. London: General Medical Council.

Heywood, L., Gonczi. A. & Hager, P. (1992). *A Guide to Development of Competency Standards for Professions*. National Office of Overseas Skills Recognition Research Paper No. 7. Canberra: Australian Government Publishing Service.

Hubbard, J. P. (1971). *Measuring Medical Education*. Philadelphia: Lea & Febiger.

Hubbard, J. P., Levit, E. J., Schumacher, C. G. & Schnabel, T. G. (1965). An objective evaluation of clinical competence. *New England Journal of Medicine*, **272**, 1321–8.

Lazarus, J. H., Baum, M. & Kilpatrick, G. S. (1976). The final examination in the United Kingdom medical schools, 1974. *Medical Education*, **10**, 109–12.

Newble, D. I. & Swanson, D. B. (1988). Psychometric characteristics of the objective structured clinical examination. *Medical Education*, **22**, 325–34.

Renwick, W. L. *et al.* (1988). *The Education of Medical Undergraduates in New Zealand.* Report of the Review Committee. Wellington: Medical Council of New Zealand.

Rhodes, P. (1985). *An Outline History of Medicine.* London: Butterworth.

Stokes, J. (1974). *The Clinical Examination – Assessment of Clinical Skills.* Medical Education Booklet No. 2. Dundee: Association for the Study of Medical Education.

3

Licensure and specialty board certification in North America: background information and issues

SUSAN CASE and IAN BOWMER

Licensure in the USA

In 1992, a new licensing examination system was established in the USA. This system, the United States Medical Licensing Examination (USMLE), includes a three-step examination, each step of which must be passed for initial licensure. The USMLE replaces the two alternative examination systems for allopathic medical practitioners. All doctors who seek a license to practice medicine in the USA, regardless of whether they were educated in the USA or elsewhere, are required to pass the USMLE. Although licenses are granted by individual legislative jurisdictions, the USMLE is required uniformly.

Typically, Step 1 is taken by students at the end of their second year of medical school following two years of basic science education. The purpose of Step 1 is to assess whether an examinee understands and can apply key concepts of basic biomedical science. The test includes approximately 700 multiple-choice questions (MCQs). The majority of items assess application of basic science principles to clinical situations, interpretation of pictorial or tabular material, and other 'problem solving' skills; many are posed within the context of a patient vignette.

Usually, Step 2 is taken by students during their fourth year of medical school. The purpose of Step 2 is to assess whether an examinee possesses the medical knowledge and understanding of clinical science considered to be essential for the provision of patient care under supervision. Step 2 also includes approximately 700 MCQs. Questions focus on content that is important for any new graduate to know, regardless of area of specialization.

Step 3 is designed to be taken during the first year of postgraduate education. The purpose of Step 3 is to assess whether an examinee possesses the medical knowledge and understanding of biomedical and

19

clinical science considered to be essential for the unsupervised practice of medicine. Questions on this examination focus on managing patients, including health maintenance, clinical interventions, clinical therapeutics, and legal/ethical and health care systems.

Step 1 and Step 2 were implemented in 1992 and Step 3 will be phased in during 1994.

Question format

Despite continued debate about the appropriateness of multiple-choice tests, all three Step examinations currently include only MCQs. In a quest for the optimal evaluation instrument, the National Board of Medical Examiners (NBME) has conducted continual research on test formats. For the past 20 years, a major focus of this research has been the computer based examination (CBX) project (Clyman & Orr, 1990; Melnick, 1990). Since the mid-1970s, a second area of research has focused on standardized patients (SPs). While both the CBX and the SP projects are in a research mode currently, both are being considered for use in Step 2. As with other forms of more 'authentic assessment', CBX and SP-based examinations appear to provide significant advantages over MCQ tests for assessment of clinical competence: they have good face validity and pose tasks for the examinee in a way that may appear to be more realistic than MCQs. However, there are psychometric and practical problems that require better solutions before these methods can be used for licensure in the USA (Millman, 1991; Hambleton & Murphy, 1992; Kane, 1992).

While these research projects continue, other projects have focused on enhancing the multiple-choice format. As a result of test development research, MCQs today appear very different from those used in the past. For content, as well as psychometric reasons, true–false varieties are no longer used on the licensure exam (Grosse & Wright, 1985; Case & Downing, 1989), and, while most of the one-best-answer questions have the traditional five options, a new format, extended matching, has as many as 26 options, pushing the examinee task to something closer to uncued free-response (Case & Swanson, 1993). In both formats, item stems are often longer and include more complete patient vignettes. Five-option items are sometimes combined into item sets which include several questions related to the same patient scenario. These include some of the advantages of simulations, while avoiding some of the disadvantages.

Test construction

The test development process for USMLE is more complex than for most examinations administered in medical schools. Questions for the licensing examination are written by content experts who serve on test committees. When these individuals are selected, care is taken to ensure that test committee members include an appropriate mix of individuals, widely representing geographical regions, medical schools and personal demographic variables. Committee members serve a limited term to maintain turnover.

Each item writer is taught how to construct MCQs, usually in a two-day workshop. Individuals write questions on assigned topics, and send them to the NBME for review and evaluation by test development staff. Annotated questions are then reviewed and approved in a test committee meeting, during which each question is read aloud and critiqued by other members of the committee. As an additional quality control mechanism, questions from each committee are reviewed and approved in a meeting of the Chairs of the individual committees. Finally, items that have been approved by the Chairs are generally pretested within an unscored section of the examination before being used as 'live' (i.e. scored) items.

An extensive (30 page) content outline guides the content of each examination. An oversight committee meets periodically to approve each examination and to approve any changes proposed for the content outline. The content outline, plus sample items, is available to the medical school faculty and to individuals registered to take the examination. However, the allocations of items for each content area (i.e. the content weights) are not provided.

There are several tensions that influence the construction of each Step examination. As dictated by the purpose statements noted above, the USMLE is designed for general licensure; it is not an achievement test. Step 2, for example, is designed to assess the application of knowledge required for beginning the first postmedical school year, regardless of specialty. The focus on content that is necessary for practice, rather than explicitly on content that has been taught (if it were possible to catalog such a body of information), means that questions might be included that are not taught uniformly in medical school. In contrast, it is possible that topics taught in some medical schools might be omitted from the examination. In reality, there is a close association between what is taught in medical school and what is included on the examination, but the examination is designed to be an independent assessment of what students need to know, regardless of whether or not it is taught. To avoid dictating the curriculum of individual medical schools, while at the same time providing necessary information about the examinations to examinees, the general content outline (without content weights) is published.

A second tension arises from the focus on knowledge that is required by the general undifferentiated doctor. Critics question the appropriateness of a general examination in an era of specialization. However, a general, rather than a specialty-specific, license is received and this is believed to give a mandate that the examination be general. This debate continues into the specialty board certification arena, as is noted below.

Standard setting

Pass–fail standards for the Step examinations are now based on content review of examination materials, supplemented by information on the previous performance of examinees and on surveys of various constituents about appropriate failure rates. Following establishment of this standard, it has been equated forward, ensuring that subsequent examinees are held to the same standard as those on the original administration (Swanson *et al.*, 1991). Provision is made to review the standard annually and to undertake in-depth analysis and review every three years.

Specialty Board certification in the USA

Following licensure, most physicians continue graduate medical education (residency training) and seek certification from a specialty board. Unlike licensure, certification is not required by law. However, hospitals may require specialty board certification as a prerequisite for obtaining certain privileges. The American Board of Medical Specialties (ABMS) is an association, currently of 24 member boards, founded to assist its members in their efforts to evaluate and certify specialists. The first specialty board in the USA (Ophthalmology) was founded in 1917. Other boards founded by the late 1930s include internal medicine, obstetrics and gynecology, orthopaedic surgery, otolaryngology, pathology, pediatrics, psychiatry, radiology, surgery, and urology; 14 other boards have become members since then. In addition to ABMS boards, there are over 120 'self-designated boards' not recognized by the ABMS.

ABMS specialty board certification is sought by most current medical school graduates, although there is no professional or legal requirement for a medical practitioner to obtain it. All 24 boards require applicants to pass a written MCQ examination to obtain certification. Over half the boards (generally the smaller ones) also require candidates to pass an oral examination. As an illustration, the following section provides a description of the examination programme of the American Board of Orthopaedic Surgery (ABOS).

Certifying examinations of the American Board of Orthopaedic Surgery

The ABOS requires candidates to have graduated from medical school, to have passed the licensure examination and to have completed five years of graduate training in the specialty before sitting for the six-hour written examination. This examination includes 300 MCQs in either a standard five-option or extended matching format. It is viewed as a certifying examination for the general orthopaedic surgeon, regardless of subspecialty. Most questions are based on a patient vignette with associated pictorial material. The questions require the examinee to select the most likely diagnosis or the most appropriate next step in patient care. The test development process is similar to that noted above for the licensure examination.

Candidates who have passed the written examination, and have completed two years of specialty practice, can sit for the oral examination. This two-hour examination contains three parts: one of the examiners concentrates primarily on six oral cases, with protocols developed by the examination committee; another concentrates on records of ten cases brought from the candidate's practice; and the third concentrates on a submitted list of all patients treated by the candidate over a six-month period. These examiners provide independent ratings on the components and then meet to establish an overall pass–fail determination. Provision is made for reexamination by a second team of examiners if the first team is unable to arrive at a pass–fail decision or if a reexamination is requested by the examinee.

Since 1986, individuals who have passed the written and oral examinations have become 'board certified' in orthopaedics. This certification expires after 10 years.

Specialization

The issue of specialization is undergoing considerable debate in the USA for both licensure and certification examinations at all levels. Most medical students begin to specialize while still in medical school with specialization becoming increasingly narrow during residency training. Yet specialty boards often regard their certificate as indicating general certification in the specialty, thus requiring assessment of skills across the breadth of the specialty.

Licensure in Canada

Background

In Canada, the authority to grant a license to practice medicine rests in the hands of the provinces and is delegated to provincial medical boards. These exist under acts of the provincial legislatures and are empowered to define competence and ensure that competence is maintained to an accepted standard. Since 1912, the Medical Council of Canada has been responsible for establishing a qualification in the practice of medicine acceptable to these licensing authorities. The Canada Medical Act of 1912 not only established the council but also defined its role in conducting the examination process (Kerr, 1979). Until recent years, measurable competencies of the practicing doctor were not explicit but were implicit in the process of developing the examination content. Panels of content experts in the different areas of medicine wrote the questions. Scoring was the duty of the examiner and standard setting was the duty of the examination committee.

With the new assessment methods of the 1950s and 1960s, essay questions and oral examinations were abandoned and, in 1965, objective, machine-marked examinations were introduced. Content was determined by new test committees established from what were considered the core specialty disciplines of medicine, surgery, psychiatry, obstetrics and gynecology, pediatrics, public health and preventive medicine. Standards were ensured not through established objectives but through the composition of the test committees. Specialists, general practitioners, educators and community-based practitioners from across the country developed the questions based on their perception of contemporary Canadian medicine. The standard was based on the performance of a reference group of Canadian medical students. The score that failed four per cent of the reference group was adopted as the passing score for all candidates.

In 1976, the Act was amended to confirm the Council's role in research and development in the evaluation of medical knowledge and clinical competency (Kerr, 1979). Standing committees were established to include this area, as were committees for education, legislation, finance and appeals. By 1982, Council had also recognized the need to assess the non-cognitive abilities of the medical practitioner (McClure, 1982).

Current procedures

Beginning in 1984, task forces of individuals from across the country were established to develop objectives for the examination process. These objectives gave credence to a belief, already voiced in Council, that the multiple-choice examination did not effectively assess clinical decision-making, bedside clinical skills, technical skills or attitudes. Concerns were also expressed about the use of patient management problems. The First Cambridge Conference recognized that such patient management problems, introduced to assess clinical decision-making, had very poor reliability (Norman *et al.*, 1985). Alternative formats were developed and, based on these, a proposal was submitted to the Council to develop a paper examination to assess decision-making utilizing the recognition of 'key features' in clinical problems (Bordage & Page, 1987). The licensing authorities, who comprise almost two-thirds of the Council, also formally requested examinations of clinical skills and attitudes. The development of a multi-station national clinical examination was pilot-tested in February 1991 for introduction in November 1992. Standard setting for the Council's examinations was also reviewed and criterion-referenced (content-based) standard-setting techniques were adopted, to be introduced into all examination processes by 1992.

The result of these endeavors has been a significantly revised evaluation process. The multiple-choice component of the examination has been completely reviewed and revised by the test committees, based on an examination blueprint derived from the new objectives. The patient management problems were reduced in 1991 and completely replaced in 1992 with the new 'key feature' clinical decision-making questions. Bordage & Page (1987) have demonstrated that these questions have high face and content validity and are reliable in the context of the current examination. Finally, the Council approved the development of an entirely new multi-station objective structured clinical examination (OSCE) format to assess clinical skills and attitudes, the so-called Q5 examination.

Entrance to the new examination, the Qualifying Examination Part I (QE-I), requires the candidate to be either in the final year, or a graduate, of a Liaison Committee on Medical Education or Committee on Accreditation of Canadian Medical Schools (LCME/CACMS) accredited medical school or a graduate of a medical school listed in the World Health Organization (WHO) directory, with successful completion of the Medical Council evaluating examination. Entrance to the Qualifying Examination Part II (Q5 or QE-II) requires successful completion of the Part I examination and 12 months of postgraduate education. Licensure in Canada will be awarded without further training to all individuals who have passed Part I and Part II, that is those who are Licentiates of the Medical Council of Canada and who received certification from either the College of Family Physicians or the Royal College of Physicians and Surgeons of Canada. By 1993 all provinces except Quebec will require the components of the Licentiate but may give licenses without certification if provincially determined postgraduate education requirements are met.

References

Bordage, G. & Page, G. (1987). An alternative approach to PMPs: the 'key features' concept. In *Further Developments in Assessing Clinical Competence*, ed. I. R. Hart & R. M. Harden, pp. 59–72. Montreal: Can Heal Publications.

Case, S. M. & Downing, S. M. (1989). Performance of various multiple-choice item types on medical specialty examinations: types A, B, C, K, and X. In *Proceedings of Twenty-Eighth Annual Conference on Research in Medical Education*, pp. 167–72. Washington: Association of American Medical Colleges.

Case, S. M. & Swanson, D. B. (1993). Extended matching: a practical alternative to free-response questions. *Teaching and Learning in Medicine*, **5**, 107–15.

Clyman, S. G. & Orr, N. A. (1990). Status report on the NBME's computer-based testing. *Academic Medicine*, **65**, 235–41.

Grosse, M. E. & Wright, B. D. (1985). Validity and reliability of true-false tests. *Educational and Psychological Measurement*, **45**, 1–13.

Hambleton, R. K. & Murphy, E. (1992). A psychometric perspective on authentic measurement. *Applied Measurement in Education*, **5**, 1–16.

Kane, M. T. (1992). The assessment of professional competence. *Evaluation and the Health Professions*, **15**, 163–82.

Kerr, R. B. (1979). *History of the Medical Council of Canada*. Victoria BC: Morris Printing Co. Ltd.

McClure, W. (1982). *Assessing Non-Cognitive Skills*. Report to the Medical Council of Canada.

Melnick, D. E. (1990). Computer-based clinical simulations: state of the art. *Evaluation & the Health Professions*, **13**, 104–20.

Millman, J. (1991). Teacher licensing and the new assessment methodologies. *Applied Measurement in Education*, **4**, 363–70.

Norman, G. R., Bordage, G., Curry, L., Dauphinee, D., Jolly, B., Newble, D., Rothman, A., Stalenhoef, B. M., Stillman, P., Swanson, D. & Tonesk, X. (1985). A review of recent innovations in assessments. In *Directions in Clinical Assessment*, ed. R. E. Wakeford, pp. 9–27. Cambridge: Cambridge University School of Clinical Medicine.

Swanson, D., Case, S., Kelley, P., Lawley, J., Nungester, R., Powell, R. & Volle, R. (1991). Phase-in of the NBME comprehensive Part I examination. *Academic Medicine*, **66**, 443–4.

4

Issues in recertification in North America

JOHN NORCINI and BETH DAWSON-SAUNDERS

The credentialing process

In order to practice, a physician in North America must have graduated from an accredited medical school and must obtain a license to practice. The license itself is unrestricted, in other words a doctor may practice in any field and may use the title of specialist upon merely holding a valid license. The desire on the part of some practitioners to establish their credentials as specialists prompted them to develop a voluntary certification process based on meeting well-defined standards. Credentialing consists of three components: accreditation, licensure and specialty certification.

Accreditation of undergraduate medical educational programmes in both the USA and Canada follows identical guidelines, thus establishing one standard for medical education in North America. In both countries, it is accomplished by a joint accreditation committee of the national medical association and the national medical college association, a procedure described in detail in Chapter 3. Graduate education in the USA is overseen by residency review committees and councils of the American Medical Association (AMA); in Canada, it is one of the responsibilities of two organizations, the Royal College of Physicians and Surgeons of Canada (RCPSC) and the College of Family Physicians of Canada (CFPC).

Individual states or provinces have the legal authority to license practitioners (and other health care professionals), generally coordinating their activities through voluntary membership of national associations (e.g. the Federation of State Medical Boards in the USA, the Federation of Provincial Medical Licensing Associations in Canada). The requirements for licensure typically include:

(i) Graduation from an accredited USA or Canadian medical school, or a special certification process for graduates from medical schools not in North America (administered by the Educational Commission on Foreign Medical Graduates in the USA and by the Medical Council of Canada in Canada)
(ii) A period of supervised graduate education in an approved internship or residency programme, often lasting one year
(iii) Passing a national examination. After a phase-in programme beginning in 1991, there will be one national examination programme only in the USA (the United States Medical Licensing Examination). In Canada, most provinces require passage of the Medical Council of Canada licensure examination

Generally, there is reciprocity of licensure among states within the USA and within the provinces of Canada. Reciprocity between the two countries is more complicated and depends on the state and province involved. At the present time, the license is awarded for life so long as the practitioner performs according to certain codes of conduct. However, at least one state has proposed requiring periodic recredentialing (Gellhorn, 1991).

As practitioners in the USA and Canada began voluntarily to limit their practice to a specific area of medicine, they formed specialty societies and boards and developed formal training programmes. Soon afterwards, the accreditation of these training programmes and the establishment or assignment of agencies to oversee formal assessment procedures was undertaken in order to ensure the quality of the graduates. In the USA, as of 1991, there were 23 specialty boards that certify doctors in various specialties and subspecialties. They coordinate their activities through the American Board of Medical Specialties (ABMS) in order to maintain high standards and to oversee the establishment of additional specialties and/or subspecialties. In Canada, licensure is under the auspices of the provincial councils and specialty certification functions are under those of the RCPSC and the CFPC.

Recertification

In the USA, members of the maturing specialty boards considered the issue of maintaining standards through voluntary recertification and time-limited certification (Lloyd & Langsley, 1987; Benson, 1991; Gellhorn, 1991; Langsley, 1991). The term 'time-limited', as used in this chapter, refers to a process in which the certificate awarded is valid only for a given period of time. Although the issue of recertification has been the subject of discussion among Canadian physicians, in Canada, the role of voluntary education is emphasized and compulsory recertification is not required currently.

There were a number of reasons for interest in methods to maintain standards, including the growing and changing body of medical knowledge and the need for accountability. In the USA, some of the forces working toward recertification include:

(i)   The profession's desire for excellence and recognition
(ii) Increasing public interest and awareness
(iii) The possibility of governmental legislation (Chase & Burg, 1987).

The American Board of Internal Medicine (ABIM) gave the first recertification examination in 1974 on a voluntary basis, but enrollment decreased subsequently (Langdon *et al.*, 1989). When established in 1969, the American Board of Family Practice instituted time-limited certification requiring subsequent recertification (also time-limited). By 1991, 16 of the 23 specialty boards either had instituted or had plans to institute time-limited certification/recertification (Annual Report and Reference Handbook, 1991). A listing of the boards, the year in which time-limited recertification was or is to be implemented, the duration of their certificates, and examination requirements are given in Table 4.1.

The remainder of this chapter contains a discussion of various issues in recertification and ends with comments on the evaluation of the recertification process itself.

Goals of recertification

Benson (1991) had identified four goals of a recertification process that would fulfill the need for accountability. By holding practitioners to a standard throughout their careers, he suggests that the profession would achieve the following goals: (i) improve patient care; (ii) set standards for the practice of medicine; (iii) foster learning throughout a lifetime; and (iv) reassure the public, including legislative bodies, by identifying the incompetent practitioner.

Reasons for and against time-limited certification

A number of arguments for time-limited recertification have been put forward. Benson (1991, p. 238) points out that 'professional accountability requires a self-regulating profession to set and maintain credible,

Table 4.1. *American specialty boards and recertification requirements*

American Board of examination	Year began	Time limit	CME	Maintenance of licensure	Performance evaluation	Written examination
Allergy/immunology	1989	10	No	?	No	Yes
Anesthesiology	—					
Colon/rectal surgery	1990[a]	8	Yes	Yes	?	Yes
Dermatology	1991[a]	10	Yes	Yes	?	Yes
Emergency medicine	1980	10	No	Yes	?	Yes[b]
Family medicine	1969	7	Yes	Yes	Yes	Yes
Internal medicine	1990	10	No	Yes	Yes	Yes
Neurological surgery	—					
Nuclear medicine	1992[a]	10	No	Yes	?	Yes
Obstetrics/gynecology	1986	10	No	Yes	Yes	Yes
Ophthalmology	1992[a]	10	?	?	?	?
Orthopaedic surgery	1986	10	Yes	Yes	Yes	Yes[b]
Otolaryngology	1989[c]					
Pathology	1979[c]					
Pediatrics	1988	7	No	Yes	No	Yes
Phys med/rehabilitation	1993[a]	10	?	Yes	?	?
Plastic surgery	?					
Preventive medicine	—					
Psychiatry/neurology	1991[a,d]	10	?	Yes	?	?
Radiology	—					
Surgery	1976[e]	10	Yes	Yes	Yes	Yes
Thoracic surgery	1976	10	Yes	No	Yes	Yes[f]
Urology	1985	10	Yes	Yes	Yes	Yes[f]

CME is continuing medical education.
— means boards without recertification programmes.
? means policy was not formulated, as of 1991.
[a] Year proposed to begin; not all requirements firmly established.
[b] One of the pathways currently available.
[c] Recertification is not time-limited.
[d] 1991 for General psychiatry; 1994 for all other psychiatry/neurology areas.
[e] 1975 for Pediatric surgery.
[f] Self-assessment (take-home) examination.
Adapted from Tables 3, 4 and 7 in Lloyd (1987) and from Table 6 in *Annual Report and Reference Handbook* (1991).

useful standards for its members' and by enforcing its own standards maintains its integrity. Thus, recertification provides the opportunity for the profession to continue to improve the quality of medical care.

Jaffe & Berg (1987) discuss five advantages of time-limited certification. They suggest that:

(i) It induces self-evaluation by requiring doctors to document their competence
(ii) It promotes self-improvement by encouraging doctors to keep up-to-date with progress in the field, to take courses, etc.

(iii) It results in collective improvement of the entire profession as a result of individual improvement
(iv) It causes the profession to take a leadership role in setting standards for the practice of medicine
(v) It keeps the body of knowledge intact by reducing splintering and fragmentation

Arguments may also be made that recertification helps to protect the public by ensuring that diplomates have retained, as well as attained, a standard of excellence and that the recertification process will focus increased energy on the problems related to the measurement of clinical competence.

Several authors (e.g. Jaffe & Berg, 1987; Stevens, 1987) provide insight into why there has been some resistance to time-limited certification. The most cogent argument is that it cannot be done properly. Opponents to recertification claim that most programmes are based on tests of knowledge, not tests of what actually happens in practice, and that there has been limited research indicating the predictive validity of such examinations. Consequently, they believe that a significant price is paid by those who fail to be recertified by this flawed process and that society may be deprived of a practitioner who is functioning at an acceptable level. However, several boards attempt to assess components of competence other than knowledge (see 'Components of an ideal recertification programme' below) and more studies of the predictive validity of certification examinations are under way (e.g. Hartz *et al.*, 1989; Ramsey *et al.*, 1989).

A second argument from those who oppose time-limited certification avers that practitioners improve throughout their careers. From this perspective, the constant interaction with patients increases procedural, technical and humanistic skills while improving clinical judgement, the most important aspect of clinical competence. Proponents of this perspective acknowledge that there is a rapidly expanding knowledge base, but suggest that mandating continuing medical education would be a more reasonable means of ensuring that doctors are up-to-date. They claim that a recertifying process would be time-consuming and unproductive, since it would extend to areas beyond the scope of particular practices.

The third, and final, argument against time-limited certification cites lack of support among practicing doctors and some specialty societies. It also suggests that the expectations of the public are unreasonable and that some of the external pressures from legislators and third-party payers have shifted to cost-containment that is less related to demonstration of on-going competence.

Eligibility requirements

Eligibility requirements for recertification, by definition, must include initial certification in the relevant specialty. However, boards vary in their requirement of whether or not the certificate, if time-limited, must be valid at the time of attempted recertification. Boards may choose to impose some requirements for candidates whose previous time-limited certificate has expired prior to becoming recertified, such as passing a 'qualifying' examination prior to admittance to the recertification process.

Several of the USA specialty boards require maintenance of a valid license for recertification (see Table 4.1). Practitioners may be ineligible for recertification if they have been subject to disciplinary actions by licensing bodies and their licenses have been withdrawn or restricted, and/or if they have lost hospital privileges because of impairment, malpractice, or other reasons. Since recertification is a continuing pathway to practice, it must attest to the continuing moral and ethical standing of the doctor. This process is facilitated by the recent establishment of a national data base of disciplinary actions taken by licensing bodies. Some boards may wish to reserve the right to limit the acceptance of candidates in such circumstances (e.g. Glassock *et al.*, 1991).

Content of the recertification process

Focus

The content of examinations for time-limited recertification can be based on cutting-edge knowledge or current practice. The assumption underlying a focus on cutting-edge information is that stable medical knowledge does not decay, even if it is not in use as part of practice. Consequently, physicians need only acquire information that has changed since their last assessment. However, a test composed of cutting-edge knowledge is potentially less relevant because some of the information may never have a bearing on practice. On the other hand, it would probably encourage more study, since candidates for recertification are likely to know less of this information. For the same reason, such a test would also be perceived as more threatening by practitioners.

Content focused on current practice does not make an assumption about whether medical knowledge decays over time. Instead, the content of the test seeks to represent practice. Obviously, such a test would be more relevant than a test of cutting-edge knowledge but it would encourage less preparation. It would also be less threatening to practitioners.

Breadth

The content of the test can be so broad that it covers the entire domain of the certificate, or it can be tailored to the practice of the candidate. There are good reasons to devise a recertification programme that assesses both.

Holding a license or certificate implies competence in a relatively broad domain. A medical license permits a practitioner to provide virtually any kind of medical or surgical treatment. Since most practitioners tend to specialize in an area, a tailored assessment of practice alone is insufficient to ensure competence in the broader field. Consequently, recertification must attest to potential in these areas.

On the other hand, an assessment that is tailored to practice is probably the most attractive form of evaluation for both the public and the practitioners. To the public, recertification would provide direct evidence that the practitioners are or are not achieving appropriate results given what they actually do. To the practitioners, this type of assessment offers the opportunity to be judged on their day-to-day activities.

Level

The content of a recertification programme can be targeted to the level of the generalist, specialist, or subspecialist as appropriate. A more complicated issue is whether the specialist and subspecialist will be held accountable for general content. As with the issue of breadth of content, it could be argued that an assessment that is limited to the level of practice is most attractive from the standpoint of both the public and the practitioners.

Nevertheless there is some justification for requiring that all specialists and subspecialists are familiar with a core of general information. Such content is encountered in even the most subspecialized practices. Moreover, provision of general care is a large component of the practice of some specialists. Finally, integration of general information into specialty and subspecialty assessment ensures that entire disciplines remain intact rather than becoming fragmented.

Duration of the certificate

Once a specialty board has decided to limit the duration of the certificate, several other issues must be resolved. All USA specialty boards instituting time-limited certification have opted for it to take effect with a specific starting date for all subsequent diplomates, but those already certified retain their lifetime certification. However, it is possible, at least theoretically, to implement a time-limited certification programme that would require all those certified currently to recertify as well.

A primary consideration is the length of time a certificate remains valid. The times chosen by various specialty boards vary between seven and ten years, sometimes supported by the claim that the half-life of a medical fact is seven years (Langsley, 1987). It is important that the duration should be neither too short nor too long but, within a reasonable range, the choice is somewhat arbitrary.

Another issue is whether the duration of the certificate is of fixed or variable length. For example, the Board of Family Practice and the Board of Pediatrics award certificates for a fixed length of time (seven years) and most diplomates take the recertification examination only one year prior to the expiration of their certificate. The American Board of Internal Medicine awards certificates for ten years and diplomates may begin the recertification programme at any time during this period. If successful, they are recertified for 10 years from the date of completion.

The number of times a diplomate may attempt to recertify may range from a specific number, such as the three attempts permitted by the ABIM, to an unlimited number of attempts, as permitted by the American Board of Surgery. All specialty boards in the USA allow at least one retake of the examination.

The action that boards choose to take for diplomates who are not successful in the recertification process may also vary. Many have concluded that some type of action is necessary 'to put teeth' into the process. For example, ABIM diplomates with time-limited certification who opt not to recertify or who are unsuccessful in their attempts will no longer be listed as 'board-certified' in various directories such as the Directory of Medical Specialties or the ABMS Compendium of Certified Medical Specialists (Glassock *et al.*, 1991). As with practitioners who permit their time-limited certification to expire, those who have been unsuccessful in their attempts to recertify may wish, at a future date, to reestablish their eligibility for recertification. In such circumstances boards can be expected to specify criteria for reentry into the recertification process for these candidates.

Boards that award certification in subspecialty areas usually require diplomates to be certified in the general specialty (e.g. internal medicine) before they are eligible to be become certified in a subspecialty (e.g. oncology, cardiology or rheumatology). A question that then arises is whether recertification in a subspecialty area implies recertification in the general area as well. The Board of Pediatrics has resolved this issue in the affirmative by designing a 'core' portion of each subspecialty examination devoted to general pediatrics. The ABIM, on the other hand, requires the diplomate who wishes to maintain certification in general internal medicine as well as in a subspecialty to pass both examinations. However, some activities and some examination components fulfill requirements for both certificates.

Setting standards

There are several methods for setting standards and much has been written in the measurement literature on the topic (see Chapter 15; Livingston & Zieky, 1982). An important issue for recertification is whether candidates should be held to the same standards as those for initial certification. From the perspective of the public, it seems reasonable to expect a doctor to maintain the same level of competence, regardless of age or time since training. Standards must be equivalent for a board's certificate to have the same meaning over a practitioner's career.

Despite these arguments, standards for initial certification and recertification are often different. Studies have shown a decrement in performance on most written examinations starting 10 to 15 years after training (Norcini *et al.*, 1985). This decrement may be caused by a failure of candidates to keep abreast of changes in knowledge or the questions in the examinations may become less relevant to mature practice. Regardless of the cause, boards are reluctant to fail large numbers of the older candidates and consequently they change the standards.

One way to avoid this problem is to allow candidates to tailor the content of the examination (within limits) to their practices, perhaps by using a modular format. Items within each module could be chosen so that they are relevant to practice (see Chapter 13). Under such circumstances, decrements in performance are less likely and when they occur are more often due to the failure of candidates to keep up with changes in medical knowledge. Consequently, smaller pass rates are easier to justify.

Continuing medical education

Formal continuing medical education (CME) courses provide one mechanism for meeting the goal of promoting lifelong learning among doctors. Twenty-three states in the USA currently require the completion of specific amounts of CME. However, there is little evidence that this requirement has a major effect on the way doctors practice or on the choice of courses important to their clinical practice (Davis *et al.*, 1990). Thus, it has been questioned whether CME alone provides sufficiently for maintaining competence.

Some specialty boards require CME as one of several components of their recertification process (see Table 4.1). The relationship between CME and recertification is especially close in Pediatrics in which a self-assessment examination is available each year and a journal is published (*Pediatrics in Review*) containing educational materials related to the objectives tested by the recertification examination (Brownlee, 1987). The ABIM recertification examination has no formal linkage to CME (Benson, 1991). However, candidates will receive prompt feedback on the diagnostic assessment component of the recertification programme that should help them to choose areas in which to focus educational efforts.

Whether CME is formally linked to the recertification examination or indirectly related through feedback on self-assessment exercises, the amount of detail provided to candidates needs to be considered. An overly large amount of detail may promote candidates to 'study to the test', clearly not a desirable outcome. Conversely, feedback that is too vague is not very useful in identifying a pattern of strengths and weaknesses. Feedback for areas of weakness must contain sufficient detail for candidates to know where their knowledge is deficient.

Components of an ideal recertification programme

The assessments used in recertification or relicensure programmes should provide a complete picture of the competence of the practitioner and should have three components. First, the programme should warrant the competence of the doctor as demonstrated in actual practice and this could be achieved by an assessment of patient outcomes. Second, the recertification programme should warrant that a practitioner has the potential to respond appropriately to a wide range of problems that are not seen routinely in practice, and this could be addressed in an assessment of the candidate's knowledge base with an emphasis on recent advances and rare but important occurrences. Third, recertification should warrant the interpersonal and moral characteristics of the practitioner by a credentials review and by collecting the opinions of peers and patients.

First component

In many ways, patient outcomes are the ultimate criterion providing a direct measure of the consequences of what is actually done in practice, thus avoiding many of the problems associated with traditional measures of competence (Relman, 1988). Many of the conventional measures are one or more steps removed from practice and reflect the potential to perform rather than the actual performance. In addition, it is difficult to tailor the content of recertification examinations to the varied and unique practices of the individual examinees using current methods of assessment. Outcomes assessment, on the other hand, permits recertification in what practitioners actually do in their professional activities rather than in the total discipline.

Patient outcomes have been used as a criterion in medical research for quite some time. Most common are studies that compare patient outcomes for two or more different treatments of the same medical condition. These studies have traditionally concentrated on mortality and morbidity as the end points of interest. More recent work has broadened the definition of outcomes so that it includes other important clinical end points such as the functional status of patients, patient satisfaction, and cost effectiveness (Kaplan, *et al.*, 1988; Lohr, 1988, 1990; Wennberg, 1988). Similarly, the range of factors influencing outcomes has been expanded to include those such as the characteristics of the health care system and the health care provider.

As promising as this technology is, outcomes assessment is still in its infancy and has some serious limitations (Epstein, 1990). First, the vast majority of the research has been done in a hospital setting where patients are acutely ill or particular procedures are involved (e.g. surgery). In these situations, appropriate outcomes can be relatively clearly defined. In contrast, the bulk of medical practice is in an ambulatory setting where problems are chronic, good outcomes are difficult to define and significant follow-up is required to document an effect.

Second, the activity of a medical practitioner is rarely the sole reason for any particular outcome. Whether a patient gets better is often more a function of the patient's problem and the initial severity of the condition. The patient's willingness and ability to comply with the doctor's orders, the resources available to the doctor, the performance of other members of the health care team, and a host of other factors also contribute.

Finally, virtually all work in this area has been done with a large number of physicians on a limited number of conditions. This has allowed collection of enough cases on a single topic to permit good analyses and adjustment for factors, other than the doctor, that affect outcomes. For evaluation of the individual practitioner, considerable work remains.

Until the gap between ideal and practical methods of assessing outcomes is narrowed, Kremer (1991 p. 193) has recommended that 'process measures known to correlate with patient outcomes could serve as standards for judging physician performance in recertification programs'. In other words, the process of care that a practitioner provides to a patient could be used to evaluate actual performance in practice. However, the process on which the practitioner is judged must be demonstrated empirically to have an association with patients' outcomes.

Standards for the process of each condition could be derived by reviewing experimental evidence or by consensus of a panel of experts (Kremer, 1991). In a publication by the Institute of Medicine, Lohr (1990) suggests a four-step process for developing quality-of-care criteria. First, a thorough review of the literature is undertaken, using meta-analytic techniques as appropriate and desirable. Second, a group of experts is convened to review the literature and to develop the criteria (i.e. answer key). Third, the criteria are pilot tested, and, fourth, the impact on patient care is monitored.

Outside of the surgical specialties, at least two medical certifying boards have experience with methods that form the basis for meaningful outcomes-related process measures. As one part of its recertification process, the American Board of Emergency Medicine has offered chart stimulated recall since 1987 (Munger & Reinhart, 1987; Solomon *et al.*, 1990). The examinee submits the medical records of six consecutive cases to the Board. Two oral examiners then select three of the six cases and, in a face-to-face interaction, question the examinee in an effort to assess the diagnosis and management of the case. Information in the chart, supplemented by interaction between the examiners and examinee, permits modification of the criteria (i.e. answer key) when dictated by the particulars of the case (e.g. severity of disease, patient compliance). This process could be made even better if the Board developed explicit criteria and sampled cases more broadly for the individual practitioner.

As part of its time-limited certification programme, the American Board of Family Practice has a computerized chart audit (Leigh, 1987). The Board asks for three medical charts for each of three different medical conditions (e.g. hypertension, diabetes mellitus, urinary tract infection). The charts are selected by the physician who provides a summary of each on machine readable forms. These summaries are judged against criteria established by consensus of the Board. To encourage accurate recording, the Board occasionally asks for photocopies of the original medical records, and Board representatives routinely visit and inspect the charts of a certain percentage of examinees. Examinees are informed how their performance relates to that of their colleagues and whether they fall below Board standards on the criteria. Among the currently used methods, this comes closest to fulfilling the requirements of a process-related outcome measure.

Second component

Beyond the routine aspects of practice that can be assessed by patient outcomes, there are facets of competence that are important and encountered infrequently or are relatively new developments. Consequently, the second component of an ideal recertification programme is an assessment of potential to practice.

The goal of this component of recertification is to ensure that the practitioner is able to respond appropriately to those cases or situations that are important, new, or encountered infrequently. There are two aspects in achieving this goal: First, a well-designed recertification process should encourage practitioners to learn, or relearn, how to handle as many of these cases or situations as possible using the best methods currently available in their discipline. In other words, it should set in motion a process of continuous improvement. Second, the process needs to warrant that the practitioner has met certain minimum standards, thus protecting the public. To achieve these two ends, a two-part examination is necessary. The first part should provide the examinee with diagnostic information that corresponds in some obvious way to formal and informal continuing education. The second part should provide a summative decision about the potential to practice.

Diagnostic evaluation

The purpose of diagnostic testing is to stimulate continuous improvement by providing practitioners with a measure of their potential to diagnose and to treat important but infrequent diseases and, more broadly, to be cognizant of recent medical advances. To fulfill these purposes, the test(s) should possess three characteristics: questions must be relevant to clinical practice even if the topic is new or emerging; the method of testing should permit very broad sampling of the content in an efficient fashion; and feedback should be specific and linked in some apparent way to education.

Among the testing methods currently available, very few have all the characteristics of a good diagnostic test. However, the need for relevant test material posed in the context of a clinical situation provides an advantage to those methods of assessment that simulate the physician–patient interaction. From lowest to highest fidelity, options ranged from using patient-based multiple-choice questions that assess higher order aspects of competence to using standardized patients and oral examinations (see Chapter 1; Lloyd, 1983). Between these two extremes are a host of written, computer-based and video simulations, as well as models, heart sound machines and the like. Among the methods, patient-based multiple-choice questions provide a reasonable alternative for large-scale evaluation, given current testing limitations. They lack the face validity of other measures, but they permit very broad sampling in a reasonable amount of testing time and the feedback can be very specific and linked to education. Multiple-choice questions used for such a purpose must stress higher-order cognitive skills and avoid the 'simple recall of knowledge' that has, unfortunately, characterized the use of this format.

Summative evaluation

The purpose of a summative test is to protect the public by warranting that the practitioner has met certain minimum standards. For credibility, the test questions should focus on aspects of medicine that are relevant to the diagnosis and treatment of patients, and posed within the context of a particular patient problem. This ensures that an examinee's performance will more likely generalize to the real clinical situation.

There are three important ways in which a summative examination differs from a diagnostic examination. First, given the need to protect the public, a summative test must be administered in a secure environment. With today's technology, that typically means a proctored examination with confidential test material. Second, the purpose of examination feedback will be to convey some sense of overall performance rather than specific information on performances in content areas. Third, because it is not necessary to identify areas of particular strength or weakness, the item formats used for summative tests do not need to be quite as efficient as the formats used for diagnostic tests.

Among the testing methods currently available, many would be suitable as summative measures of cognitive ability. As with diagnostic tests, the need for relevant test material presented in a clinical setting gives an edge to the methods of assessment that simulate the physician–patient interaction.

Third Component

The third component of recertification provides an assessment of the nontechnical facets of competence. Specifically, it reassures the profession and the public that the practitioner behaves in a moral and ethical manner, is not impaired and has reasonable relationships with patients.

In order to achieve the goals of this component of a recertification process, information is needed from credentialing authorities, colleagues and patients. The purpose of collecting credentialing information is to establish the moral and ethical characteristics of the practitioner and to determine whether impairment is a problem. The data can come from several sources. First, information on disciplinary actions by licensing bodies should be reviewed prior to recertification. This information has been assembled recently in the USA through the establishment of a national database to permit the unscrupulous practitioner to be tracked across state boundaries. Second, data from local credentialing bodies, such as hospitals, should be reviewed. Third, because there are legitimate reasons why such information would not be available (e.g. a physician may not have hospital privileges), alternative forms of evaluation should be pursued. For example, statements about the physician's moral and ethical standing in the community could be sought from local authorities.

Collection of data from colleagues and patients can provide an assessment of the interpersonal relationship between the practitioner and the patient. At this time, the most practical method for gathering such information is the collection of ratings. Recent work used the ratings of patients to gauge their satisfaction with the interpersonal aspects of care (Swanson *et al.*, 1990). Ratings from 30 to 50 patients were required to obtain a stable estimate of an individual physician. Work by Butterfield & Pearsol (1990) with ratings of nurses yielded similar results. Ramsey and colleagues have shown that ratings of professional qualities obtained from medical colleagues identified by the practitioner yielded reasonable results with 10 to 20 ratings and differentiated between internists who were and were not certified (Carline *et al.*, 1989; Ramsey *et al.*, 1990).

Evaluation of the recertification process

As with any high-stakes assessment, the validity of tests used as part of the recertification programme should be established using well-accepted procedures (e.g. the *Standards for Educational and Psychological Testing*, 1985). Regardless of the focus and breadth of the content, it must be relevant to practitioners and should represent the knowledge and skills that practitioners use or need in their daily work. Expected relationships between performance on the test and other measures of clinical competence should be evaluated in formal validity studies.

The goals of recertification are laudable and, if successfully met, can be expected to have a measurable impact upon the quality of medical care. Tests themselves constitute only one of three components of an ideal recertification programme. Establishing the validity of these tests, while important, does not establish the validity of the entire recertification programme itself. More is needed. The guidelines for developing process-related outcome measures discussed above, if followed properly, promote validity inherently through the manner in which the criteria are established. The assessment of the non-technical facets of competence also needs to be carried out using valid (and reliable) procedures. The evaluation of how successfully all three components of the recertification programme are developed and executed should be part of establishing the validity of the recertification process itself. Evidence in favor of the validity of recertification will accrue if the indicators of the quality of medical care respond in the expected directions. Specifying the degree of impact a comprehensive recertification programme should have on traditional indicators is important in designing good validity studies and in keeping expectations for the programme reasonable.

References

Annual Report and Reference Handbook (1991). Evanston: American Board of Medical Specialties.

Benson, J. A., Jr (1991). Certification and recertification: one approach to professional accountability. *Annals of Internal Medicine*, **114**, 238–42.

Brownlee, R. C. (1987). Recertification examinations linked to CME. In *Recertification for Medical Specialists*, ed. J. S. Lloyd & D. G. Langsley, pp. 43–8. Evanston: American Board of Medical Specialties.

Butterfield, P. S. & Pearsol, J. A. (1990). Nurses in resident evaluation: a qualitative study of the participants perspectives. *Evaluation and the Health Professions*, **13**, 453–73.

Carline, J. D., Wenrich, M. & Ramsey, P. G. (1989). Characteristics of ratings of physician competence by professional associates. *Evaluation and the Health Professions*, **12**, 409–13.

Chase, R. A. & Burg, F. D. (1987). Reexamination/recertification: measurement of professional competence and relation to quality of medical care. In *Recertification for Medical Specialists*, ed. J. S. Lloyd & D. G. Langsley, pp. 141–7. Evanston: American Board of Medical Specialties.

Davis, D. A., Norman, G. R., Painvin, A., Lindsay, E., Ragheer, M. S. & Rath, D. (1990). Attempting to ensure physician competence. *Journal of the American Medical Association*, **263**, 2041–2.

Epstein, A. M. (1990). The outcomes movement – will it get us where we want to go? *New England Journal of Medicine*, **323**, 266–70.

Gellhorn, A. (1991). Periodic physician recredentialing. *Journal of the American Medical Association*, **265**, 752–5.

Glassock, R. J., Benson, J. A., Jr, Copeland, R. B., Godwin, H. G. Jr, Johanson, W. G. Jr, Point, W., Popp, R. L., Scherr, L., Stein, J. H. & Taunton, O. D. (1991). Time-limited certification and recertification: the program of the American Board of Internal Medicine. The task force on recertification. *Annals of Internal Medicine*, **114**, 59–62.

Hartz, A. J., Krakauer, H., Kuhn, E. M., Young, M., Jacobsen, S. J., Gay, G., Muenz, L., Katzoff, M., Bailey, R. C. & Rimm, A. A. (1989). Hospital characteristics and mortality rates. *New England Journal of Medicine*, **321**, 1720–5.

Jaffe, B. M. & Berg, L. (1987). Pros and cons of time-limited certification. In *Recertification for Medical Specialists*, ed. J. S. Lloyd & D. G. Langsley, pp. 59–67. Evanston: American Board of Medical Specialties.

Kaplan, S. H., Greenfield, S. & Ware, J. E. Jr (1988). Assessing the effects of physician–patient interactions on the outcomes of chronic disease. *Medical Care*, **27**, S110–27.

Kremer, B. K. (1991). Physician recertification and outcomes assessment. *Evaluation and the Health Professions*, **14**, 187–200.

Langdon, L. O., Grosso, L. J., Glassock, R. J., Copeland, R. B. & Kimball, H. R. (1989). Advanced achievement in internal medicine: the end of the line for voluntary recertification. *The Journal of General Internal Medicine*, **4**, 557–9.

Langsley, D. G. (1987). Prior ABMS conferences on recertification. In *Recertification for Medical Specialists*, ed. J. S. Lloyd & D. G. Langsley, pp. 11–27. Evanston: American Board of Medical Specialties.

Langsley, D. G. (1991). Recredentialing. *Journal of the American Medical Association*, **265**, 772.

Leigh, T. M. (1987). Computerized office record review. In *Recertification for Medical Specialists*, ed. J. S. Lloyd & D. G. Langsley, pp. 103–20. Evanston: American Board of Medical Specialties.

Livingston, S. A. & Zieky, M. J. (1982). *Passing Scores: A Manual for Setting Standards of Performance on Educational and Occupational Tests*. Princeton: Educational Testing Service.

Lloyd, J. S. (Ed.) (1983). *Oral Examinations in Medical Specialty Board Certification*. Evanston: American Board of Medical Specialties.

Lloyd, J. S. (1987). History and present status of recertification. In *Recertification for Medical Specialists*, ed. J. S. Lloyd & D. G. Langsley, pp. 3–9. Evanston: American Board of Medical Specialties.

Lloyd, J. S. & Langsley, D. G. (Eds.) (1987). *Recertification for Medical Specialists*. Evanston: American Board of Medical Specialties.

Lohr, K. N. (1988). Outcome measurement: concepts and questions. *Inquiry*, **25**, 37–50.

Lohr, K. N. (Ed.) (1990). *Medicare: A Strategy for Quality Assurance*. Washington: National Academy Press.

Munger, B. S. & Reinhart, M. A. (1987). Field trial of multiple recertification methods. In *Recertification for Medical Specialists*, ed. J. S. Lloyd & D. G. Langsley, pp. 71–88. Evanston: American Board of Medical Specialties.

Norcini, J. J., Lipner, R. S., Benson, J. A. & Webster, G. D. (1985). An analysis of the knowledge base of practicing internists as measured by the 1980 recertification examination. *Annals of Internal Medicine*, **102**, 385–9.

Ramsey, P. G., Carline, J. D., Inui, T. S., Larson, E. B., LoGerfo, J. P. & Wenrich, M. D. (1989). Predictive validity of certification by the American Board of Internal Medicine. *Annals of Internal Medicine*, **110**, 719–26.

Ramsey, P. G., Carline, J. D., Inui, T. S., Larson, E. B., LoGerfo, J. P. & Wenrich, M. D. (1990). *Assessment of the clinical competence of certified internists* (Final Report). Philadelphia: American Board of Internal Medicine.

Relman, A. S. (1988). Assessment and accountability: the third revolution in medical care. *New England Journal of Medicine*, **319**, 1220–2.

Solomon, D. J., Reinhart, M. A., Bridgham, R. G., Munger, B. S. & Starnaman, S. (1990). An assessment of an oral examination format for evaluating clinical competence in emergency medicine. *Academic Medicine*, **65**, S43–4.

Standards for Educational and Psychological Testing (1985). Washington: American Psychological Association.

Stevens, W. C. (1987). Why we decided not to recertify. In *Recertification for Medical Specialists*, ed. J. S. Lloyd & D. G. Langsley, pp. 55–8. Evanston: American Board of Medical Specialties.

Swanson, D. B., Webster, G. D. & Norcini, J. J. (1990). Precision of patient ratings of residents' humanistic qualities: how many items and patients are enough? In *Teaching and Assessing Clinical Competence*, ed. W. Bender, R. Hiemstra, A. J. J. A. Scherpbier & R. Zwierstra, pp. 424–31. Groningen: BoekWerk Publications.

Wennberg, J. E. (1988). Outcomes research, cost containment, and the fear of health care rationing. *New England Journal of Medicine*, **323**, 1202–4.

5

Recertification: an Australasian perspective

ROGER GABB

In Australia, a practising specialist is required to have either certification as a Fellow of an Australian college or an approved specialist qualification from another country. Responsibility for registration (licensure) of medical practitioners rests with State and Territory Governments, which have established medical boards or their equivalent to adminster this process. Most States maintain a single register for all medical practitioners while two states operate a separate register for specialists. All, however, restrict the use of the term 'specialist' to those medical practitioners with approved specialist qualifications.

In the early 1970s, the Federal Government introduced a national health scheme. Under this scheme, provision was made for the payment of medical benefits (in the form of a partial reimbursement of patient fees) at higher rates for services provided by specialists. Because most states did not maintain a separate register of specialists, the Federal Government then set up a mechanism to determine which practitioners should be recognized as specialists and thus be eligible for higher fee rebates under the national health scheme. For this purpose, Specialist Recognition Advisory Committees were set up in each State or Territory to determine whether individual practitioners should be recognized as specialists. A national body, the National Specialist Qualification Advisory Committee (NSQAC), was then established to provide uniform guidance to these state registration and recognition bodies on which specialist medical qualifications should be accepted. The general principle on which NSQAC operates is that registration or recognition of a specialist is based on the completion of a programme of appropriate supervised training covering a minimum of six years after medical graduation and an examination leading to the award of a higher qualification. The qualification must be awarded by, or equate to that awarded

47

by, the relevant specialist professional college in Australia (NSQAC, 1990).

This general principle uses the duration of training for the local qualification as an important criterion and, because the period of training required by Australian colleges is longer than that required in most other countries, a relatively small number of recognized qualifications is listed for each accepted specialty. In obstetrics and gynaecology, for example, only four (non-subspecialist) qualifications are listed as 'appropriate'. These are Fellowship of the Royal Australian College of Obstetricians and Gynaecologists (FRACOG), Fellowship (under certain conditions) of the Royal New Zealand College of Obstetricians and Gynaecologists (FRNZCOG) and Fellowship or Membership (under certain conditions) of the Royal College of Obstetricians and Gynaecologists (FRCOG or MRCOG). The list is somewhat longer in other specialties, such as internal medicine and surgery.

From the above, it will be clear that the Australian colleges have considerable power in controlling who can practise as a specialist in Australia. Like their counterparts in the United Kingdom, the Australian colleges are pluripotent organizations. Like their sister colleges in the United States of America, they have responsibility for continuing medical education (CME) and other matters directly affecting their Fellows but they also carry responsibility for accreditation of training posts and training programmes in hospitals and for conducting certification examinations. Thus, they perform functions associated in the USA with both the Specialty Boards and the Accreditation Council for Graduate Medical Education (and its Residency Review Committees).

This integration of functions within a single organization has some obvious advantages in terms of coordination within the continuum of medical education. It also has some potential disadvantages. Benson (1991) claims that a major strength of the American Board of Internal Medicine is that it has no constituency and thus can be true to its mission of certifying excellence in the specialty. If this claim can be substantiated, there is potentially a conflict of interest in Australian colleges because those who determine the entrance requirements are the same people who look after the interests of those already in the specialty group. What is certain, however, is that in Australia the responsibility for ensuring high standards in a specialty rests very largely with a single organization. That organization is therefore in a position to implement a coordinated range of strategies aimed at maintaining the standard of service provided by its Fellows.

One other matter deserves some explanation. Australia and New Zealand are two independent countries separated by the Tasman Sea (and much else besides!). The situation described above is found in Australia and should not be construed as applying to New Zealand as well. However, most clinical colleges in Australia are actually Australasian in that they draw their membership from practitioners in both countries (e.g. Royal *Australasian* College of Surgeons (RACS), Royal *Australian and New Zealand* College of Psychiatrists (RANZCP). In a few cases, separate Australian and New Zealand colleges exist (e.g. in general practice and obstetrics/gynaecology).

Maintaining standards

Every college has as one of its stated aims the maintenance of professional standards. The majority claim that maintaining standards is the most important of their aims and that all others are secondary to this overarching aim. The term 'maintaining standards' is, of course, a convenient shorthand term for something more than the static conservation of the existing standards of professional practice that it suggests. It is concerned with ensuring that the quality of service offered by the members of the college reflects the growing body of knowledge associated with that specialty. It is, therefore, a dynamic concept associated with improving as well as maintaining standards. Used in this way, it is concerned with maintaining the highest standards of professional service consistent with the current body of knowledge associated with that specialty.

Before examining some of the issues relating to recertification in Australia, it seems sensible to reflect on why colleges should be concerned with the maintenance of standards. There appear to be three main arguments supporting the involvement of a college in maintaining the standards of professional practice and these are discussed below.

Public interest

The community implicitly grants an Australian college a considerable amount of power. In effect, most of the power to determine who can practise as a specialist in Australia resides in the college. In return, the community charges the college implicitly with responsibility for maintaining standards in that specialty. Given its power, the college has a moral obligation to ensure that the community is provided with a high standard of care in the discipline. The notion of autonomy linked to self-regulation lies at the very heart of the professional ideal.

Long-term self-interest

It is, of course, in the long-term interest of a college and its Fellows to maintain standards within a specialty. The long-term standing of the specialty depends on the quality of service offered by its practitioners. All members benefit to some degree when a professional group is seen as having high standards and all members suffer to some degree when some members of the group are shown publicly to have low standards. So, not only is it in the interests of the community for the college to concern itself with standards, but also it is in the interests of the Fellows themselves.

Short-term self-interest

This is best encapsulated in the frequently heard argument: 'If we don't do it to ourselves, someone else will do it to us!' This is a defensive reason for maintaining standards. It assumes that 'someone else' (often assumed to be a government instrumentality) would be less benevolent and less understanding in dealing with maintenance of standards than the college itself.

Each of these arguments is cogent in its own way. Colleges must concern themselves with the maintenance of standards. A college which does not do so effectively deserves to be labelled as self-serving rather than self-regulating and to have its standing in the community reduced accordingly.

Strategies for maintaining standards

There are two main categories of strategy used by Australian colleges – entry strategies and maintenance strategies. There is also a third group of strategies not considered here which might be called environmental strategies, whereby the college attempts to influence the environment in which the service is provided in order to ensure that high standards are maintained. These strategies are sometimes aimed at maintaining working conditions or levels of remuneration and this industrial flavour makes them somewhat controversial.

Entry strategies are used commonly by colleges to maintain standards. These focus on the accreditation of training and certification of new entrants to the profession. The Royal Australian College of Obstetricians and Gynaecologists (RACOG), for example, is involved in the selection of new trainees, accreditation of training programmes in hospitals, provision of postgraduate courses and certification of trainees first as Members (an interim qualification) and then as Fellows of the College. Each of these is a strategy for maintaining standards in the profession by ensuring that new members of the professional group are competent.

As well as entry strategies, most colleges also employ strategies aimed at maintaining high standards of service by those already admitted to the professional group. The following strategies are either used by Australian colleges or, at least, theoretically available to them:

(i) Setting standards of professional practice – the college determines and promulgates ethical and technical standards of service

(ii) Informing Fellows of professional development activities – the college keeps its Fellows informed of both continuing education activities and other professional development activities, such as quality assurance programmes

(iii) Accrediting professional development activities – the college not only informs its Fellows of professional development activities but also approves activities offered by other providers

(iv) Providing professional development activities – the college develops a range of professional development activities for its Fellows

(v) Withdrawing certification from Fellows who fail to meet professional standards – the college may withdraw Fellowship or certification from a Fellow because of a gross failure to maintain ethical or technical standards

The remainder of the strategies listed here involve recertification, i.e. the college requires its Fellows periodically to meet certain criteria as a condition of continuing full Fellowship. True recertification involves time-limited certification, in which a certificate of Fellowship expires after a predetermined period (say, 10 years) and its renewal for a further defined period is contingent on the Fellow meeting certain college requirements.

(vi) Recertification based on continuing professional experience – the college requires Fellows to submit evidence of their continuing

      involvement in professional activity, documenting a certain num-
      ber of hours of professional practice per year, for example
(vii) Recertification based on participation in professional development
      activities – the college requires its Fellows to document their
      participation in professional development activities
(viii) Recertification based on assessment of competence – the college
      requires its Fellows to undergo periodic tests of competence or
      capability such as tests of clinical knowledge, tests of clinical
      judgement or tests of surgical skill
(ix)   Recertification based on assessment of performance – the college
      requires its Fellows to provide evidence of their professional
      performance. Thus, a doctor might be asked to provide authenti-
      cated medical records of all cases seen over a certain period and
      these might be assessed in order to evaluate his or her mode of
      practice
(x)   Recertification based on assessment of outcomes – rather than
      assessing the performance itself, the college assesses the outcome
      of professional performance

Some of these maintenance strategies might be characterized as 'negative' because they are aimed at reducing the prevalence of substandard
care. Strategies such as withdrawing certification because of major
deficiencies in professional performance or withholding recertification
because of major deficiencies identified in a recertification examination
are instances of negative strategies. These strategies are based on what
Berwick (1989) calls the 'Theory of Bad Apples'. They are negative not in
any pejorative sense but simply because their prime focus is on the
detection and remediation of instances of substandard care. Most colleges in Australia have the power to use such negative strategies, even if
they exercise it infrequently. Some colleges, such as the RACS and the
RANZCP, have strengthened their disciplinary procedures recently so
that they can deal more effectively with complaints about the performance of their Fellows from other Fellows, other health professionals,
hospitals and consumers.

While agreeing that there is a place for such negative strategies to deal
with those providing grossly deficient care, Berwick (1989) argues for a
stronger emphasis on 'positive' strategies, those based on what he calls
the 'Theory of Continuous Improvement'. As he describes them, these
strategies focus on encouraging continuous improvement by the average
practitioner and not on identifying and dealing with outliers. Such

approaches assume, probably correctly, that most Fellows provide care of a high standard already and are committed to continuous improvement. All colleges in Australia and New Zealand already employ a range of positive strategies aimed at encouraging their Fellows to improve their standards of care continually. These include promulgation of practice guidelines, provision of continuing education activities and, more recently, the support of quality assurance activities at a local level. Indeed, most colleges are more active in their use of such positive strategies than in the use of negative strategies based on the identification of substandard care.

Some of these strategies can be seen as purely positive or purely negative while most have both positive and negative elements. Some strategies are aimed primarily at increasing the general competence of the membership and only incidentally at the detection and remediation of outliers. A strategy linking recertification to involvement in effective professional development activities, for example, might be expected to increase the general level of competence in the professional community without necessarily decreasing the incidence of individual acts of gross incompetence, which are commonly caused by factors other than deficiencies in knowledge or skill. Similarly, a recertification strategy based on regular assessment of clinical performance by means of practice audit may have as its primary aim the detection of individuals who are providing poor quality care, although it may also stimulate practitioners to improve their standard of care both because of the threat of audit and by providing them with useful feedback on their learning needs.

Recertification

There are several arguments for the use of recertification as a strategy for maintaining professional standards. In many Australian colleges, there is a gross imbalance between entry strategies and maintenance strategies. A common pattern is to have strong, rigorously enforced entry strategies and weak, unenforced maintenance strategies. It is difficult to convince community critics that this arrangement is designed to protect their interests. Often they conclude, perhaps rightly, that the Fellows of such colleges are more concerned with looking after themselves than in guarding the interests of the community at large. In other words, these colleges appear to be more interested in self-service than in self-regulation.

Weak maintenance strategies are disadvantageous to the professional group as well. Every professional community has at least a few members who fail to maintain high standards of practice because they are too busy, do not see it as a high priority or suffer some form of impairment which reduces their effectiveness. The threatened sanctions of a recertification strategy may be one way of 'encouraging' these practitioners to raise the standard of their professional practice.

Finally, it seems likely that the ideal of the autonomous professional group will survive only if colleges are seen to be genuinely self-regulating. There is, in the community at large, a general disenchantment with the professions. Today's community is sceptical of the claims of professionals and demands much more accountability than it ever did previously. As Relman (1988) has pointed out, medicine has moved through two revolutionary eras, the 'Era of Expansion' and the 'Era of Cost Containment', and is now in the 'Era of Assessment and Accountability'. Genuine self-regulation, which will include some form of recertification, is the only approach which will prevent or, at least, postpone more regulation of professional activity from outside the profession.

Deciding on which recertification strategy to adopt is a complex problem, as the whole issue of recertification is strongly political. In judging the soundness of a strategy, it is therefore necessary to take into account factors other than the technical soundness (reliability, validity, generalizability, etc.) of the method used. The experience of the RACOG in introducing its recertification programme suggests that at least four main factors need to be considered. These are its effectiveness in maintaining standards, how feasible it would be to implement, its acceptability to the Fellows of the College and its credibility to the community at large.

Assessing the potential effectiveness of a strategy is a difficult task. In the first place, it is necessary to be clear about what the strategy is designed to achieve. As noted above, it may be that the main objective is the positive one of ensuring continuous improvement in the care provided by the Fellows of the college. On the other hand, the objective may be the negative one of decreasing the incidence of individual acts of incompetence by Fellows of the college. In other words, the impact of the strategy may be judged either by changes in the overall quality of care offered by the professional community or by changes in the incidence of substandard care.

The feasibility of a recertification strategy is determined largely by its demands on the college. In introducing a recertification strategy, the college needs to consider the financial cost of its introduction as well as the human resources it will require. This includes a consideration of both the demands it will make on Fellows of the college and the need for staff members with the appropriate skills and expertise. For example, a college considering a recertification scheme based on practice audit needs to assess the considerable resource implications of such a scheme. A Canadian programmes of practice audit, for example, was costed in 1984 as $786 (Canadian) per practitioner (McAuley, 1988). In general terms, programmes based on documentation of participation in professional development activities or a pencil-and-paper examination can be expected to be considerably less costly than a programme of periodic performance-based assessment.

Because a recertification programme is something which the Fellows of a college impose on themselves, the acceptability of the strategy to Fellows is a crucial consideration. In the first place, it is necessary to consider how much the strategy might cost individual Fellows. This must include the direct cost to the Fellows, in terms of increased subscription or recertification fees to support these activities and, perhaps, the cost of increased participation in professional development activities. In addition, the indirect cost of reducing the incomes of Fellows while they are engaged in non-income-generating activities required for recertification must also be considered.

It is also important that the strategy is seen by Fellows as being fair. This means that no subgroup of Fellows can be seen as being particularly advantaged or disadvantaged by the strategy. Thus, it must be equally applicable to generalists and subspecialists, metropolitan practitioners and non-metropolitan practitioners, academics and non-academics, private practitioners and those receiving a salary, and so on. Associated with the concept of fairness is that of punitiveness. The threat of sanctions in the form of withdrawal of Fellowship or certification by the college is necessarily a part of a recertification scheme. A strategy is likely to be more acceptable to the Fellows of a college if the sanctions are applied firmly and fairly but in a manner which is seen by Fellows as non-Draconian. Finally, a strategy is more likely to be acceptable to Fellows if it is seen clearly as protecting patient confidentiality. Any strategy which requires the disclosure of confidential information about patients to the college is likely to have relatively low acceptability.

Recertification strategies are often implemented because of real or imagined community pressure for a greater degree of demonstrable accountability. For this reason, the credibility of the recertification strategy in the eyes of the community is very important. Ideally, the strategy should not only be credible to the community at the time of its introduction, but should also maintain its credibility in the longer term. For example, recertification strategies linked to involvement in continuing education activities may be credible in Australia in 1993 but may not be acceptable to the community in 10 or 20 years' time. It is likely that tomorrow's community will demand that recertification be linked more directly to professional performance.

Recertification in Australasia

At this time, only two colleges in Australasia have functioning recertification programmes. These are the RACOG and the RNZCOG. Two other colleges, the RACS and the Royal Australasian College of Physicians (RACP) have announced that they will introduce recertification in the near future. Other specialist colleges, such as the Royal Australian College of Ophthalmologists, are considering the concept actively (Murchland, 1988) and some have surveyed their members to establish their attitudes to recertification. Other major colleges, such as the RANZCP have declared their opposition to the notion of recertification (RANZCP, 1989).

The current situation of the Royal Australian College of General Practitioners (RACGP) is somewhat complex. The College does not operate a recertification scheme based on time-limited certification but its members are expected to participate in some of the professional development activities of the College's 'Quality Assurance Programme'. Recently, however, the Federal Government has introduced a 'Vocational Register of General Practitioners'. Vocational registration qualifies the practitioner for somewhat higher levels of patient rebate from the Health Insurance Commission. It is not necessary to be a Fellow of the RACGP to maintain one's place on the Vocational Register but one must participate in RACGP-approved quality assurance activities at a level identical to that required for continuing membership of the RACGP. Thus, somewhat paradoxically, even though the College itself does not operate a recertification system based on time-limited certification for its own members, it services a Government scheme which is, in effect, based on time-limited registration.

The Royal Australian College of Obstetricians and Gynaecologists (RACOG)

The recertification programme developed by the RACOG has become a model for several other Colleges in Australasia and, indeed, in other countries including the UK and Canada. It will, therefore, be described in some detail.

The RACOG introduced time-limited Fellowship at the time of its foundation in 1978. Up until that time, those wishing to obtain specialist qualifications in obstetrics and gynaecology in Australia did so through the Australian Regional Council of the British Royal College of Obstetricians and Gynaecologists (RCOG). All Fellows of the RACOG, from the 500 or so Foundation Fellows who were 'grandfathered' into the College on the basis of their (mostly) British qualifications to the most recently elevated Fellow in 1993, are granted their Fellowship initially for a 10-year period. Then, providing they meet recertification requirements, they are granted further five-year extensions of their Fellowship.

The College's 'Continuing Education/Continuing Certification' programme is a form of recertification linked to involvement in professional development activities. Recertification is based on the accumulation, over a five-year period, of 150 cognate points (based on one point per hour of involvement) for participation in a range of professional development activities. In the initial 10-year Fellowship period, these activities must take place in the last five years of that period while activities can occur at any time during subsequent five-year recertification periods.

Approved professional development activities fall into five categories discussed below, with points maxima defined in all categories (RACOG, 1989).

(i)   Educator activities – this category includes: publication of papers and books; presentation of papers at meetings; and teaching students and registrars. A total of 60 points can be earned for educator activities

(ii) Attendance at CME meetings – this includes attendance at congresses, courses, conferences and workshops organized both by the College and by other providers. While a maximum of 30 points can be earned by attending non-approved meetings, such as local hospital CME meetings, most must be earned by attendance at meetings approved by the College. Proof of registration at these meetings is required. A maximum of 130 points can be earned by attending CME meetings

(iii) Supervised learning projects – Fellows may arrange their own learning experiences, typically attendance at a special unit or clinic to gain knowledge and skill in a specialized area. Supporting documentation must be submitted, including learning objectives, learning strategies used, method of assessment used and proof of attendance. A maximum of 50 points can be earned for this activity in a five-year period

(iv) Involvement in quality-assurance activities – cognate points can be earned by providing evidence of attendance at hospital quality-assurance meetings. To support this activity, the College is developing a set of clinical indicators for use as the first tier of a two-tiered quality-assurance procedure. In addition, the College organizes regional quality-assurance activities for some non-metropolitan practitioners. Up to 50 points can be claimed for documented participation in quality-assurance activities in one five-year period

(v) Completion of self-assessment tests – the college produces three different types of self-assessment test: those associated with brief clinical reviews sent to all Fellows; those associated with a subscription series of audio tapes; and a series of more comprehensive GOAL (gynaecology and obstetrics: assessment for learning) self-assessment programmes. The tests can either be submitted by mail to the College for marking and feedback or completed interactively using the College's computer bulletin board system. Points are awarded for submission of completed tests for marking and feedback rather than for achieving a certain standard. A maximum of 120 points can be earned by submitting completed self-assessment tests

Evaluating the effectiveness of this strategy is proving to be very difficult. It is clearly a strategy aimed at encouraging high levels of performance rather than at the detection and remediation of substandard performance. However, there are a number of difficulties associated with measuring the clinical performance of a group of approximately 1000 specialist obstetrician-gynaecologists. Firstly, no generally agreed set of clinical indicators exists for the assessment of the clinical performance of obstetrician-gynaecologists. Secondly, if and when such a set of indicators is developed, it will not be possible to conduct even a quasi-experimental study because no baseline data will be available. A true randomized controlled trial is, of course, out of the question. Thirdly, the logistic problems associated with the rigorous evaluation of the effectiveness of such a national strategy are formidable. Therefore, it seems most unlikely that we will be able to demonstrate the effectiveness of the strategy in terms of its impact on practitioner competence and performance, or patient health outcomes. Instead, we will have to rely on the less satisfactory indicators of participant satisfaction, measured increase in involvement in professional development activities and 'clinical impressions'. In general terms, it is likely that the effectiveness of the strategy will depend heavily on the effectiveness of the quality assurance activities and on how well the educational components selected are related to the real educational needs of the Fellow concerned.

The feasibility of the RACOG recertification strategy has been established. One of the reasons colleges choose a recertification strategy linked to participation in professional development activities is that it is administratively feasible. Recognizing that it did not have staff with the expertise to develop, implement and evaluate the proposed programme, the College employed an educationalist as its full-time Director of Education and a social scientist as its part-time Research Officer, as well as additional secretarial/administrative staff. The main administrative cost of the programme is that of supporting these members of staff.

At this stage, the acceptability of the strategy to the Fellows of the College appears to be high. Compliance is high in that 727 Fellows have so far met the College's requirements in the last three years and only six have failed to do so. Its direct cost to each Fellow last financial year was approximately $180 for the infrastructure supporting the programme as well as for continuing education materials which are supplied to all Fellows. The cost to Fellows for their involvement in professional development activities, both in terms of the direct cost of involvement and in the opportunity cost involved, has not yet been established. The increase in these costs caused by the introduction of the programme is likely to be relatively small to individual Fellows, since most were heavily involved in CME activities before the implementation of the recertification scheme.

Much effort has been made to make the recertification programme as fair as possible to all Fellows. In particular, it has been made flexible so that Fellows in different situations can put together a mix of continuing education activities suitable for their own situation. The emphasis on a distance education approach and self-assessment testing has meant that isolated Fellows can accumulate cognate points without attending a large number of CME meetings. The RACOG programme is punitive in the sense that those Fellows who do not accumulate the required number of points are reduced to Membership status (not recognized as a specialist qualification). As noted above, this has already happened to six Fellows. However, the impression gained is that most Fellows see this consequence of the programme as unpleasant but necessary. The only threat to patient confidentiality in the RACOG programme is in the regional quality assurance cooperatives but steps have been taken here to ensure that the confidentiality of patient information is protected.

One of the main reasons for the apparent acceptance of the RACOG programme by the Fellows of the College appears to be the high level of consultation with Fellows concerning its major aspects. This consultation included national workshops open to all Fellows, local working groups for specific tasks, a postal survey of all Fellows and pilot testing of elements of the programme before its implementation (Hewson, 1989).

No systematic assessment of the credibility of the programme has been undertaken. However, informal feedback suggests that both government agencies and consumer groups find the strategy credible. This is, no doubt, partly because the RACOG is the only clinical college in Australia with a fully implemented recertification programme and in that situation, any strategy looks better than no strategy at all. The long-term credibility of the programme remains to be established.

Most of the conclusions above are based on anecdotal evidence only at this stage. As noted above, it seems unlikely that we will ever be able to establish the effectiveness of the programme in 'maintaining standards', in the sense of having a demonstrable effect on the general competence or performance of our Fellows as a group. It should be noted that this is not because of specific difficulties associated with the evaluation of this type of recertification programme, but because of problems inherent in the assessment of general competence or performance as a measure of the effectiveness of any strategy. At this stage, it seems safe to say that the feasibility of the strategy has been established, it has been shown to be generally acceptable to the Fellows of the College and it appears to be credible to the community at large.

The Royal New Zealand College of Obstetricians and Gynaecologists (RNZCOG)

Like their Australian counterparts, New Zealand obstetricians and gynaecologists trained under and were certified originally by the British College. The RNZCOG was founded in 1982 and, at that time, the College elected to grant its Fellowship for 10 years in the first instance and to follow this with five-year extensions. The College's recertification strategy is dependent on participation in continuing education and quality assurance activities. Many of the activities available to Australian Fellows are also available to New Zealand Fellows under a joint Continuing Education programme. The certification programme is, in fact, an independent RNZCOG programme but it is administered by RACOG staff.

The main difference between the New Zealand programme and the Australian one, apart from some minor differences in the maximum number of points which can be earned in particular categories, is that New Zealand Fellows *must* earn a set number of points for involvement in approved quality assurance activities.

The Royal Australasian College of Surgeons (RACS)

For several years, the RACS has collected data on its Fellows' participation in continuing education activities by means of a voluntary annual questionnaire. In 1991, the Council of the RACS resolved that it would introduce a system of recertification by 1 January 1993 (Reeve, 1991). The details of the system have yet to be announced but it has been decided that recertification will be based on participation in continuing education activities, conduct of a surgical audit and credentialing by a hospital. Thus, it seems clear that recertification will be contingent on participation in professional development activities plus demonstrated acceptance by peers in at least one hospital or clinic.

The Royal Australasian College of Physicians (RACP)

The RACP is also actively developing a recertification scheme. At this stage it appears that it will be introduced at about the same time as that of the RACS. A working party has been established to develop the system, although it is understood that it will not be based on a formal examination of any type but instead may be linked to participation in professional development activities, peer assessment and practice review.

The Royal Australian and New Zealand College of Psychiatrists (RANZCP)

The RANZCP has no recertification system currently and has stated that it is opposed to the introduction of such a scheme. However, it does operate a system of recording the participation of its Fellows in CME activities. This is entirely voluntary and not linked in any way to recertification. The College currently requests its Fellows to submit an annual 'CME record' to the College for this purpose (RANZCP, 1989).

Future developments

The age of recertification (part of Relman's (1988) 'Era of Assessment and Accountability') has just dawned in Australia and New Zealand. There are also signs that this particular sun is about to rise on other parts of the former British Empire, such as Canada (RCPSC, 1990), and also in Britain itself. In a recent newsletter, the President of the RCOG announced that the Council agreed unanimously that continuing medical education should be mandatory and linked to re-accreditation, and that this in turn should be linked to specialist registration (Simmons, 1991).

It is still too early to draw conclusions about the details of the recertification strategies which the Australasian colleges will implement finally. However, there are already some pointers suggesting that they will take a somewhat different path from that chosen by most American boards. At this stage, it looks as if most Australasian colleges will link recertification to positive strategies such as participation in professional development activities rather than to negative strategies aimed at the identification and remediation of Fellows who provide substandard care. The strategies proposed or implemented so far are aligned much more to Berwick's 'Theory of Continuous Improvement' than to his 'Theory of Bad Apples' (Berwick, 1989).

Where assessment occurs as a component of the recertification process in Australia and New Zealand, it is much more likely to be by self or by a group of peers in a hospital or region than by a national formal examination. What is to be assessed is more likely to be the process or outcome of care by a quality assurance or hospital credentialing group than clinical competence by a national body. Assessment is thus more likely to be ongoing and diffuse and less likely to be a major hurdle which must be overcome every seventh or tenth year. This form of assessment is likely to be less reliable in a technical sense than a formal examination because inevitably it will vary in its implementation from group to group and time to time.

A recertification strategy which is weighted heavily in favour of encouraging participation in professional development activities cannot be expected to perform the task of identifying and dealing with those who do not reach minimum standards. The colleges implementing such a strategy must accept therefore that practitioners who fail to obtain recertification will do so because they do not satisfy the college's requirements and not necessarily because their clinical performance is poor. In refusing to recertify a Fellow, the college will in effect be saying to that person: 'If you are unwilling to prove to us that you are committed to continuous improvement, we do not want you as a member of our group'. It cannot say legitimately: 'We do not want you as a member of our group because your clinical performance does not meet our minimum standards'. The Australasian colleges presently seem to believe that the problem of substandard practice can be addressed most efficiently by improving existing mechanisms for dealing with complaints about the performance of their Fellows.

Why have the Australasian colleges elected to implement a model of recertification which omits formal assessment of competence and which emphasizes participation in continuing education and quality assurance activities? One reason may be that many Fellows in Australia and New Zealand distrust formal examinations as a means of assessing clinical competence. This opinion may be based, at least in part, on their memories of the examinations they themselves passed many years ago; examinations which may have had limited direct relevance to their current clinical practice and which seemed somewhat arbitrary in determining those who passed. Others may recognize that certification examinations have improved considerably since then but still have reservations, like Manning & Petit (1987), that the forms of formal examination which are feasible for use with hundreds or thousands of candidates can only begin to address the assessment of competence for recertification.

Another answer may lie in the difference between the functions of the American boards and the Australasian colleges. The boards were established primarily to conduct examinations and they have become highly skilled in the business of formal assessment. For the colleges, assessment is just one of the many strategies they use for maintaining standards. Conducting the college examinations is an important task in the college year but it is only one task in a constant round of organizing continuing education meetings, negotiations with government and other agencies, servicing the needs of Fellows, organizing courses for trainees (residents), supporting quality assurance activities, etc. Therefore, these other activities are perhaps more likely to be included as elements of a recertification programme by an Australasian college than by an American board.

It may also be that the acceptability of the recertification strategy to its Fellows is of a higher priority to an Australasian college than is the acceptability of that strategy to an American board. After all, as Benson (1991) has argued, a board has no constituency and therefore can take hard decisions without too much concern for the reaction of its certificate holders. A college in Australia and New Zealand is a professional association and therefore office bearers neglect the wishes of the members of the electorate at their political peril. It may be that presently the council members of Australasian colleges judge that recertification based in part on a formal examination would be unacceptable to their constituents. Positive strategies with an emphasis on participation in college-organized or college-approved activities are much more congruent with the collegiate culture than negative strategies aimed at identifying substandard practice.

Another possible factor is that the stakes involved in recertification are potentially higher in Australia and New Zealand than they are in the United States. Failure to recertify in the United States does not prevent a practitioner from practising his or her specialty, although it may limit the opportunities for that practice. In Australia and in New Zealand, loss of Fellowship may prevent a practitioner from practising as a specialist. In New Zealand, at least, it has been suggested that the practitioner may have to undergo retraining before recommencing practice, including practice as a general practitioner. When the stakes are as high as this, a college may be less likely to opt for strategies which focus on the direct assessment of competence.

Perhaps recertification linked to participation in professional development activities is simply an important stage in the evolution of an effective recertification strategy. Practitioners in Australia and New Zealand, after all, have had no experience of relicensure based on CME credits, although many of them are well aware of some of the aberrant behaviour stimulated by that system in the USA. Therefore, no Australasian college is likely to introduce a recertification programme which relies solely on attendance at CME meetings. It is now generally accepted that, while sound educational interventions can stimulate improvement (Davis *et al.*, 1984), the number of hours of attendance at meetings is not a good predictor of performance (Davis *et al.*, 1990). Nonetheless, persuading Fellows to accept a system based on participation in continuing education activities may be an almost essential first step down the path towards a more effective system.

The ideal system of recertification must include the regular assessment of clinical performance. There are, however, two critical questions concerning the form of this assessment. The first question is whether the focus of the assessment of performance should be primarily positive (continuous improvement) or negative (substandard practice). The second is whether the locus of assessment should be national, local or something in between. In a sense, the two dominant models are those of quality assurance activities (positive, local) and formal examinations (negative, national) – the gospel according to Donabedian (1988) and the gospel according to Hubbard (1978). The developing Australasian model emphasizes the former while the current American model emphasizes the latter. However, as recent American developments (e.g. Glassock *et al.*, 1991) suggest, it may be preferable to build a system containing the best elements of both models.

References

Benson, J. A. Jr (1991). Certification and recertification: one approach to professional accountability. *Annals of Internal Medicine*, **114**, 238–42.

Berwick, D. M. (1989). Continuous improvement as an ideal in health care. *New England Journal of Medicine*. **320**, 53–6.

Davis, D., Haynes, R. B., Chambers, L., Neufeld, V. R., McGibbon, A. & Tugwell, R. (1984). The impact of CME. *Evaluation in the Health Professions*, **7**, 251–83.

Davis, D. A., Norman, G. R., Painvin, A., Lindsay, E., Ragbeer, M. S. & Rath, D. (1990). Attempting to ensure physician competence. *Journal of the American Medical Association*, **263**, 2041–2.

Donabedian, A. (1988). The quality of care. How can it be assessed? *Journal of the American Medical Association*, **260**, 1743–8.

Glassock, R. J., Benson, J. A. Jr, Copeland, R. B., Godwin, H. A. Jr, Johanson, W. G. Jr, Point, W., Popp, R. L., Scherr, L., Stein, J. H. & Taunton, O. D. (1991). Time-limited certification and recertification: the program of the American Board of Internal Medicine. *Annals of Internal Medicine*, **114**, 59–62.

Hewson, A. D. (1989). The development of the obligatory education and recertification programme of the Royal Australian College of Obstetricians and Gynaecologists: a practical response to the increasing challenges of a modern society. *Medical Teacher*, **11**, 27–37.

Hubbard, J. P. (1978). *Measuring Medical Education*. Philadelphia: Lea & Febiger.

Manning, P. R. & Petit, D. W. (1987). The past, present and future of continuing medical education. *Journal of American Medical Association*, **258**, 3542–6.

McAuley, R. G. (1988). Paper presented at the Congress on CME, Los Angeles, April 27–May 1, 1988. 'Peer review of physicians: the Ontario experience'.

Murchland, J. B. (1988). Quality assurance and recertification. *Australian and New Zealand Journal of Ophthalmology*, **16**, 255–7.

NSQAC (National Specialist Qualification Advisory Committee of Australia) (1990). *Lists of Recommended Medical Specialties and Appropriate Qualifications*. Canberra: Australian Government Publishing Service.

Reeve, T. S. (1991). President's memo. *RACS Bulletin*, **11**, 1.

Relman, A. S. (Editorial) (1988). Assessment and accountability: the third revolution in medical care. *New England Journal of Medicine*, **319**, 1220–2.

RACOG (Royal Australian College of Obstetricians and Gynaecologists) (1989). *RACOG Continuing Education Resource Manual*, Vol. 2. East Melbourne: The Royal Australian College of Obstetricians and Gynaecologists.

RANZCP (Royal Australian and New Zealand College of Psychiatrists) (1989). College position statement on CME. *RANZCP News and Notes*, **18**, 11.

RCPSC (Royal College of Physicians and Surgeons of Canada) (1990). *Maintenance of Competence System*. Ottawa: RCPSC.

Simmons, S. C. (1991). *President's newsletter*. London: Royal College of Obstetricians and Gynaecologists.

Part C

The initial certification of clinical competence

6

Guidelines for the development of effective and efficient procedures for the assessment of clinical competence

DAVID NEWBLE (Editor), DALE DAUPHINEE, BETH DAWSON-SAUNDERS, MORAG MacDONALD, HELEN MULHOLLAND, GORDON PAGE, DAVID SWANSON, ALEX THOMSON and CEES van der VLEUTEN

Additional contributors: HOWARD BARROWS, LEORA BERKSON, GEORGES BORDAGE, JANET GRANT, BRIAN JOLLY, GEOFF NORMAN, EMIL PETRUSA and REED WILLIAMS

Medical schools, medical licensing authorities and specialty certification bodies are responsible for developing procedures to assess the clinical competence of large numbers of examinees. These organizations have a history of using assessment procedures that encompass written, oral and observation-based examination formats. The performance of examinees as measured by these procedures provides the basis for decisions regarding promotion to the next stage of training, entry into medical practice and determination of hospital privileges. The decision process assumes, sometimes with little foundation, that the scores derived from the assessment procedures are a valid reflection of examinees' current level of competence and of their readiness to perform satisfactorily at the next stage of training or practice. This chapter presents a set of guidelines to assist in evaluating the validity of this risk-laden assumption.

The guidelines in this chapter are presented as a series of steps that examining bodies should follow, or be cognizant of, in developing and implementing assessment procedures. The perspective offered reflects

This Chapter is a modified version of an article previously published as Cambridge Conference Paper 7. From the Fourth Cambridge Conference, 1989.

the experiences of the authors, who have a wide range of practical and research-based expertise in the field. It also reflects a literature base that has become considerably more extensive and useful in the last few years. The chapter is not, however, an attempt to provide a comprehensive review of the literature on the assessment of clinical competence. Rather, it discusses some key issues that have not been addressed fully in reviews published elsewhere (e.g. Kane, 1982; Neufeld & Norman, 1985; Wakeford, 1985; Newble, 1992).

To make description less cumbersome the discussion will be anchored in the development of a comprehensive assessment procedure for a large class (100 or more) of medical students nearing the end of their course of studies. However, the approach we advocate can be applied equally well to the postgraduate arena.

The guidelines, which assume that the purpose of the assessment has been determined, cover the following topics:

   (i) Definition of what is to be tested
  (ii) Selection of test methods and format
 (iii) Test administration
 (iv) Test development and scoring issues
  (v) Standard setting
 (vi) Reporting scores
(vii) Item banking

Definition of what is to be tested

The most important phase in developing any assessment procedure is the definition of what is to be tested (see Chapter 7). In the terminology of testing and measurement, this guides test development and forms the basis for evaluating the content validity of the assessment procedure (Kane, 1982; Ebel, 1983; American Psychological Association *et al.*, 1985). It determines whether the procedure provides a representative and adequate sample of the competencies expected of the examinee (i.e. the graduating student). If an assessment procedure does not possess content validity, all its other attributes (e.g. face validity, reliability) are of little consequence.

The approach to determining what is to be tested consists of three steps. The first two are required to define the range of competencies that become the 'exit' or 'terminal' objectives; that is, what the student must know or be able to do at the end of the course of study. The third step is needed to identify the sample of these competencies to be tested in the assessment procedure.

Step 1: Identify the clinical problems the student should be able to handle to some level of resolution

Such problems can be identified through several approaches (see also Chapter 11). They may be generated simply by asking medical faculty to list the problems relevant to their area of specialization. If identified in this manner, the problems should be reviewed by generalists and by other specialists to ensure their applicability. A second approach is to observe and to analyse the problems and tasks to be faced by the graduates at the next stage of training: in most situations some form of internship. It is particularly important to identify those problems that a new intern is expected to deal with relatively independently.

The 'problems' may be stated in several ways. For example: they may be listed as presenting complaints, such as headache, cough or diarrhoea; or they may be phrased in the form of conditions, such as diabetes, chronic bronchitis or stroke. It may also be desirable, especially at the intern level, to include on the list of problems a range of expected practical skills, such as intravenous drip insertion, catheterization or suturing. In compiling the list, other issues that should be considered include the frequency of occurrence, the importance of early detection, the severity, and the need for immediate action at the time of patient contact (or first encounter with the problem).

Identifying the list of problems for which examinees are accountable is not a trivial task, but is more straightforward than the second step.

Step 2: For each problem, define the clinical tasks in which the examinee is expected to be competent

The term 'clinical task' has been chosen carefully to refer to actions that are specific to particular clinical problems (e.g. identifying chest pain suggestive of impending myocardial infarction, ordering laboratory studies to assess thyroid function). These tasks comprise the range of competences represented by those things the student should know or be able to do at the end of the course of study (sometimes called the 'exit' or 'terminal' objectives). If it is a patient-related problem, clinical tasks consist of all aspects of patient workup and management such as: eliciting and interpreting history (medical and psychosocial), physical examination and laboratory data; diagnosing, selecting and administering treatment; arranging follow-up; talking to relatives; and so on. If it is a public health or community-related problem, clinical tasks consist of all aspects of problem identification as well as the actions (e.g. health education, inspection of health education, inspection of health standards) that should be taken to deal with the problem.

Research on assessing clinical competence has shown repeatedly that satisfactorily fulfilling the requirements of a clinical task on one problem does not provide a basis for an accurate prediction of the ability to perform a similar task on a different problem, or even in different representations of the same problem (see Chapter 8; Swanson, 1987; Newble & Swanson, 1988; Colliver *et al.*, 1989). For example, competence in eliciting an appropriate history from a patient with chest pain may not be correlated strongly with competence in eliciting an appropriate history from a patient with acute abdominal pain. This surprising characteristic of assessing clinical competence has important consequences relating to the sampling of problems and the length of tests. These issues are discussed later in more detail.

A difficult aspect of clinical task definition is specifying the expected level of performance (see Chapter 9). At a given stage of training, some clinical tasks may be relatively trivial while others may exceed reasonable expectations. For the problem of diabetes, for example, it may be reasonable to expect a graduating student to manage a patient with controlled adult-onset type II diabetes, but it may not be reasonable to expect the same student to deal to the same degree with an adolescent with unstable type I diabetes.

When setting course objectives or curriculum development are the focus of activity, the process of defining required clinical tasks should occur ideally for each problem identified in step 1. However, for assessment purposes, clinical tasks need to be defined only for problems that have been selected for inclusion in the examination procedure, i.e. after step 3 has been completed.

Step 3: Prepare a blueprint to guide in the selection of problems to be included in the assessment procedure

Test blueprints are not new, and they come in many forms. They can be very simple and uni-dimensional, such as the percentage weight given to individual disciplines within an examination. Or, they can be complex, highly structured, multi-dimensional 'grids' in which the dimensions may reflect patient problems, organ systems, intellectual process (recall, interpretation, problem-solving), clinical setting (ward, outpatient, emergency room, community), patient age, or activities comprising the diagnostic/therapeutic process (history taking, physical examination, diagnosis, management). Blueprint dimensions should reflect an appropriate balance of health-care parameters, such as age groups and prevalence.

Although a highly structured design is not always warranted, we advocate strongly the blueprint approach to ensure that the clinical problems (and their embedded clinical tasks) contained in the assessment procedure not only are representative but also constitute an adequate sample of problems that the examinee should be capable of resolving. Such blueprints then guide the random, stratified selection of problems from the range of problems defined previously. This also ensures that subsequent test forms, constructed using the same blueprint, will assess reasonably parallel content.

Blueprints should not be used to predetermine the distribution of clinical tasks to be tested; clinical tasks must be defined in relation to the nature of the clinical problems themselves. However, the distribution of clinical tasks should be checked retrospectively to ensure a reasonable balance (e.g. to avoid over-representation of manual or therapeutic tasks relative to history taking or communication tasks). Other issues, such as the age and gender of the patient and the prevalence, severity and/or treatability of the problem, must also be taken into account when cases are being prepared to represent the selected problems.

The above approach to blueprinting a procedure for assessing clinical competence assumes the position that clinical tasks should be tested in the context of specific, relevant clinical problems and not in isolation. While there may be subcategories of clinical skills necessary for successful completion of a given clinical task, these are interrelated within any specific problem and should not be tested in isolation except, perhaps, at the early stages of clinical training. There are often many clinical tasks for any given problem, and some of them may have elements specific to the problem. The assessment procedure should be designed to test only those tasks that are most critical to the successful resolution of the problem or those that examinees will be expected to perform relatively independently in their next clinical setting. Other issues, such as selecting tasks that are expected to discriminate effectively between competent and incompetent examinees, are secondary considerations.

These three steps, although time consuming, are essential. They provide a practical and yet comprehensive approach to the identification of the 'content' to be tested through the assessment procedure. Subsequent use of elegant testing methods, computerized scoring systems and/or sophisticated analytic procedures do not compensate for the failure to define the content to be tested.

Selection of test methods and format

It is not the purpose of this chapter to discuss in detail the various test methods available for use in the assessment of clinical competence. This has been done elsewhere (see Chapter 8; Neufeld & Norman, 1985; Wakeford, 1985). Rather, the purpose is to emphasize an approach to the selection of methods based on the 'content' to be tested as defined by procedures like those outlined in the first section.

There are three issues that must be taken into account in attempting to implement the approach we advocate for selecting test methods.

Issue 1: Test methods should strive for a representation of reality (fidelity) that is appropriate to the clinical tasks being posed

For example, when the purpose of the test is limited to determining whether a student can identify the appropriate actions to take in a specific situation, such as ordering diagnostic studies, this aspect of decision making can be assessed effectively by a lower fidelity pencil-and-paper test. On the other hand, history taking or counselling tasks that require interactions with the patient are likely to require approaches of a higher fidelity, such as real or standardized-patient cases (described in more detail later).

Issue 2: The clinical task to be posed should dictate the method by which it is to be tested

This point may seem so obvious as to be unworthy of emphasis. Unfortunately, selection of assessment methods more commonly occurs first, thus determining to a large extent what is tested subsequently, without explicit consideration of the range of tasks to be posed. For example, a major reliance on multiple-choice questions (MCQ) will result in a restricted and low fidelity assessment of many clinical tasks, however high the quality of the individual test items. On the other hand, the use of clerkship ratings provided by faculty may appear to have a high index of fidelity, but may fail to assess clinical tasks involving history taking and physical examination simply because it is rare for students to be observed directly. If the need to assess such clinical tasks (e.g. taking a history from a middle-aged patient with chest pain, or conducting a neurological examination in an elderly patient complaining of paresthesia in the feet) is defined by the test blueprint, a method should be selected that entails the observation of examinees performing these tasks. This might be a rating assigned by an examiner observing the student with a real patient or a check-list completed by a trained standardized-patient. Because no assessment method is a panacea, a comprehensive assessment procedure inevitably will include more than one testing format.

Issue 3: There must be a recognition of the practical constraints on selecting optimal examination methods

It is not usually possible to achieve an ideal match between the task to be posed and the method of assessment. Constraints include:

(i) The amount of examining time available
(ii) The resources available for constructing and conducting the examination (e.g. money, examiners, organizers, patients, facilities)
(iii) The measurement characteristics of the available test methods
(iv) The acceptability of the 'ideal' approach to faculty, examinees and the profession

There is little point in designing an impractical examination procedure that could never be implemented. However, where compromises between the 'ideal' and the achievable are made these should be identified explicitly to allow improvement of the assessment procedure in the future.

Test administration

Administrative problems, such as the need to test large numbers of examinees in different examination sites or the limitations of time and other resources, have led typically to the adoption of multiple-choice-type test-methods as a major, or even the only, component of many assessment procedures. While the twin goals of efficiency and reliability are often achieved using multiple-choice tests, significant disadvantages of relying too heavily on this format have become apparent. For instance, multiple-choice tests tend to assess behaviours in isolation rather than as an integrated whole, and they are unlikely to test the full range of competencies of prime interest to the examiners. Additionally, over-reliance on their use ignores the principle that assessment will exert a strong influence on learning, potentially having undesirable effects on the approach to learning of many students (Newble & Jaeger, 1983; Frederiksen, 1984). From the same perspective, over-reliance on faculty ratings of clinical performance may cause students to limit their study to problems seen on the wards and may discourage them from reading broadly about other common and important clinical problems.

Alternative formats

Efforts have been made recently to develop more valid forms of assessment for components of clinical competence that are also more efficient and reliable than the traditional forms of clinical assessment. These efforts include pencil-and-paper and computer-based patient management problems (PMPs), the objective structured clinical examination (OSCE) and standardized patients (SPs). Each of these formats has been shown to have its limitations, one of the most frustrating being the prolonged testing time (at least 6 to 8 hours) required to achieve an acceptable level of reliability (Swanson *et al.*, 1987; Newble & Swanson, 1988; van der Vleuten & Swanson, 1990). This seems to be a phenomenon common to all methods for assessing aspects of clinical competence. It appears to be related to the inherent nature of dealing with clinical problems in which the performance on one problem is not a good predictor of performance on another (as noted above in topic 1, step 2), and it applies to the assessment of experienced physicians as well as to graduating medical students. This phenomenon has been referred to variously as 'case specificity', 'content specificity' and 'problem specificity' (Barrows *et al.*, 1978; Elstein *et al.*, 1978; Norman, 1988).

Improving efficiency of testing

It is now clear that, if we want valid and reliable assessments of clinical competence, it will be necessary to use a wider range of methods and assessment procedures that require more testing time than has been the case in the past. However, certain administrative actions can be taken to minimize the difficulty such changes would impose. An essential first step is to focus the assessment procedure on the primary need to differentiate reliably between competent and incompetent students (i.e. to make accurate pass/fail decisions), rather than to produce an equal degree of accuracy along the full scale of individual student performances for the purpose of ranking or the determination of academic honours. Such a focus leads to several possible strategies that eliminate the need for all examinees to undertake the full assessment procedure. The most promising of these is to use variable length testing procedures, such as the multiple hurdles approach, adaptive testing and sequential testing.

The multiple hurdles approach is the most readily understood of such procedures, being the one used by many postgraduate colleges and some specialty boards. This strategy is effective and efficient if the first hurdle is simple to administer (e.g. an MCQ test) and where there is a high failure rate. The second, resource-intensive hurdle (e.g. a clinical and/or oral examination) is then reached only by a subset of the examinee population. Unfortunately, the second hurdle often has the shortcoming discussed in the previous section and the final decision on examinee performance is taken on a test which is psychometrically unsound.

Another possibility is adaptive testing. When this technique is used, each component or item on the examination is selected on the basis of the examinee's performance on the previous component(s) or item(s), with the criteria for selection designed to maximize the measurement of information obtained. While theoretically sound, the complexity of the procedure means that it is most likely to be practical only in the context of computer-based assessment, and, therefore, it does not appear presently to be a realistic option for many of the testing formats used in the assessment of clinical competence (e.g. OSCE stations, standardized patients).

Sequential testing is a step toward adaptive testing, but with less complexity involved. Sequential testing is based upon the fact that, for any given test, the test length needed to make a reproducible decision about the competence of an examinee decreases as the differences between an examinee's level of competence and the pass/fail cut-off score increases. In other words, a relatively short examination may identify quite accurately those well above or well below the decision-making point. These examinees can be excused safely from further testing, and only those for whom doubt persists need to continue with a further sequence or sequences of the same examination procedure.

Sequential testing does not reduce the number of hours of testing time required for examinees near the pass/fail point. However, it does reduce the total resources required, particularly if a substantial portion of the examination involves non-written simulations. For example, an OSCE that would require three long test rotations (in parallel or on different occasions) to accommodate all students might be reduced to three shorter circuits for all students. Additional single rotations would be administered for second or third test sequences only to those students about whom doubt still exists. An important assumption of sequential testing is that each sequence, or rotation if an OSCE examination, consists of a random selection from the overall 'content' to be tested. Thus, careful attention must be paid to the preparation of the sequences (parallel forms) of the test, stratifying as appropriate for different testing formats (e.g. MCQs, OSCE stations, PMPs).

Given the desirability for assessments to move away from methods that test competencies in isolation, there must be a trend towards more comprehensive and complex procedures. Inevitably, these procedures require that more resources be allocated for testing. Since such resources are finite, it is advantageous to concentrate use where it is most needed – on those examinees close to the pass/fail point. The use of variable length testing, particularly sequential testing, seems to offer potential savings without loss of accuracy in the critical decisions that must be made. Examples of this approach can now be found in the literature, but its general acceptability has yet to be explored fully (Swanson & Norcini, 1989; Colliver, *et al.*, 1992).

Test development and scoring issues

Many issues relating to scoring have been discussed adequately in previous publications (Neufeld & Norman, 1985) and some are discussed in detail in subsequent chapters. However, since the First Cambridge Conference in 1984, certain complex test formats have been developed to increase the range and depth of the clinical and intellectual skills being evaluated and to make them a closer approximation to real-world behaviours. Examples include the written key-issue simulations (Bordage & Page, 1987) and certain forms of the OSCE station and standardized-patient-based examinations (van der Vleuten & Swanson, 1990). The comments in this section of the chapter, and those to follow on standard setting and reporting scores, focus primarily on these specific developments in testing. In these comments, the term 'case' is used to refer to a conceptual unit on the examination, whether an item or set of items on a written examination, a PMP, or a station in an OSCE-type examination.

Technical issues

There are a number of technical issues that must be addressed in the scoring of any examination. Complex clinical simulations involve additional considerations. A review of the literature provides the following guidelines (van der Vleuten & Swanson, 1990; Norman *et al.*, 1991; van der Vleuten *et al.*, 1991).

Checklists and rating scales

Both checklists and rating scales are used commonly to record performance on tests of clinical performance in which an examinee's behaviour is observed. (They may also be applicable in other contexts, such as scoring essay questions.) Checklists have demonstrated higher interrater agreement than rating scales, but the decision regarding which to use should be dictated by the skills to be tested (van der Vleuten & Swanson, 1990). It may be that both are needed (e.g. an OSCE-type examination in which one station requires an observer using a checklist to specify the actions taken by the examinee, while another station includes an assessment of the examinee's interpersonal skills supplied on a rating form completed by a standardized patient).

There has been limited research on the relationship between the length of checklists used to record actions and the reliability of the scores. Research to date suggests that longer checklists tend to be more reliable (Tamblyn, 1989). However, in some situations (e.g. standardized-patient simulations) the use of longer checklists has additional ramifications for the selection of individuals to simulate the patient problem and for the amount of time required for training. It does appear that accuracy of standardized-patient recording diminishes if more than 15 to 20 items have to be scored (Tamblyn *et al.*, 1991).

Observation and recording

Clinical assessment procedures generally require someone to observe and to record the examinee's level of performance. The observer/recorder may be faculty examiners or other trained observers. On simulations utilizing standardized patients, students may be observed and scored by the standardized patients themselves. Each approach has advantages and disadvantages (van der Vleuten & Swanson, 1990).

If standardized patients are to perform these functions, extensive training may be required. Fine distinctions and/or discriminations among specific behaviours may not be possible. The complexity of the simulation, as well as the length of the checklist or rating form, have an effect on a standardized patient's ability to remember the actions and behaviours of the examinee. Other factors, such as the length of the examination day, the number of breaks available throughout the day and the personal characteristics of the person portraying the problem, may also affect the amount of training needed.

Observation by clinical faculty examiners increases the real and hidden costs of administering the examination, although some portion of the cost is offset by reduced time for training. Faculty examiners may be able to assess more complex skills than other observers, such as the appropriateness of a sequence of information gathering or actions that have to be interpreted in a broader context. Also the observation process is beneficial to the teaching faculty by providing them with feedback, either informally or systematically, regarding the effectiveness of their teaching and the strengths and weaknesses of the curriculum. On the negative side, there is anecdotal experience to suggest that some faculty become bored by scoring checklists or rating forms, and boredom may lead to inaccuracy and unreliability.

Observers other than clinical faculty can also be used. Here, the amount of training required depends on their level of expertise. In simulations involving standardized patients, an advantage of using trained observers other than the standardized patient is their ability to record the examinee's behaviour as it occurs; they are not required to remember and to record the behaviour after the completion of the whole task performance. Before ratings by faculty and other trained observers can be assumed to be superior, their reliability as raters needs to be researched thoroughly, as has been done with ratings by standardized patients.

As with all examinations using observers, there is evidence of systematic rater bias – some are 'hawks' and some are 'doves'. This is not a problem if all students are scored by the same rater. If not, this bias can be minimized by randomly assigning students to raters within 'cases', particularly if a large number of cases is used (Tamblyn *et al.*, 1991).

Scoring keys

The use of scoring keys prepared prior to administration of the examination is a prerequisite for the efficient and timely scoring of any examination, but they are especially crucial with many of the new test developments (e.g. OSCE stations, key-issue simulations). The process of developing scoring keys a priori requires sufficient sampling of expert opinion during the preparation of the examination to ensure that the key is valid. Review of the key in the light of examinee performance after test administration is also recommended.

Weighting

Broadly speaking, weighting of items or elements within a test case, whether written or simulated, does not appear to have a major effect on the reproducibility of scores (Norcini *et al.*, 1983). Therefore, it is best to view weighting within the context of validity; that is, the weighting of elements within test cases should be guided by their importance. Weighting of content across cases should be accomplished through the design of the test blueprint rather than by weighting scores on individual cases more heavily in calculation of the total score. More important tasks should be assessed more frequently.

Case scores

Scoring on cases (e.g. PMPs, key-issue simulations, standardized patients) may be calculated as a percentage of possible points based on all elements in the case, or as an overall acceptable/unacceptable score (0–1 or pass/fail) for the entire case. The latter approach produces a total score that is less reproducible because dichotomous scoring leads to a loss of measurement information. On the other hand, the scores may be more meaningful, since they reflect acceptable performance on the cases provided in the examination more directly. However, research is extremely limited and the entire issue of how to form case scores deserves further exploration (Swanson *et al.*, 1987).

Combination of scores

The scores on cases in an examination can be combined in different ways, but the approach selected should be guided by the purpose and design of the examination (see also Chapter 10). Some educational researchers recommend designing tests so that each case, such as a single PMP or OSCE station, receives a single score. Other researchers suggest designing the test so that certain elements may be combined across cases to produce a score in a well-defined skill, such as 'history taking' or 'laboratory utilization'. The latter approach requires a high level of rigor in defining and sampling the skills to be tested. In addition, elements purported to test a specific skill should have higher correlations across cases than with elements testing other skills. To illustrate, if several cases have both history taking and laboratory utilization elements, the history taking elements should have higher correlations with each other, regardless of the case to which they belong, than with elements within the same case that test laboratory utilization.

Regardless of how the scores are formed, the test development process needs to ensure that all reported scores are both reliable and valid. Scores should not be reported on sets of elements and/or cases unless they reach an accepted level of reliability. In general, scores on individual cases do not meet those criteria and should not be reported. However, calculating scores on individual cases as a first step in computing a total score is quite acceptable. There has been no reported research on how to combine elements within cases nor research on how to combine cases themselves when tested by different formats.

Bias

Bias is known to be a potent factor in affecting student behaviour, performance and scoring (Newble & Jaeger, 1983; Frederiksen, 1984). In the context of this section, we refer to bias as a situation in which the test score has meanings or implications for a subgroup of test takers that are different from the meanings or implications for other test takers of the same ability (Cole & Moss, 1989). Although bias may be present in written tests, there are additional risks for bias in examinations involving observations of behaviour. These risks increase as the behaviour being observed becomes more difficult to define and is scored more subjectively.

There has been little research on bias and its impact on scores and on pass/fail decisions when observers are used to rate performance in real or simulated clinical situations. In particular, bias that might be related to factors such as gender and ethnicity, from the perspective of both raters and examinees, has not been investigated systematically, though reports are now appearing in the literature (Rutala *et al.*, 1991). Guidelines are needed about avoiding, monitoring, and adjusting for bias.

Equating

Equating is the process of ensuring that scores on two different tests, developed according to the same blueprint, are interchangeable (Peterson *et al.*, 1989). Equating is necessary in order to ensure comparability of scores and pass/fail decisions across multiple test forms and occasions of testing.

For written tests, a common equating method is to embed the same items (sometimes called the 'link' or 'anchor' items) within the different forms of the examination (say 30% of the total items). It is important that the anchor items represent fully the content blueprint for the entire examination. In order to equate two test forms, the performance on the anchor items is compared across the forms to estimate the relative ability of the group taking each test. The relationship between performance on the anchor items and other items within a form is then used to place scores on the same scale.

Information is scarce on appropriate methods of equating, except for those based on written tests (Skaggs & Lissitz, 1986). Equating would seem to be a difficult problem for some of the testing formats used in clinical competence assessment. Each case, rather than the elements within the case, probably should be viewed as an 'item'. With standardized patients, it may not be logistically feasible to have the same person portraying the case from one time or site to another, posing problems of equivalence. Additionally, 30% of the cases in an examination may constitute too small an absolute number of common 'items' for effective equating. At the same time, reuse of a larger number of cases may pose security problems. Limited research has been performed in this area and more is clearly needed (Rothman *et al.*, 1992).

Trivialization

Trivialization is a phenomenon to which all forms of testing are susceptible. Multiple-choice questions have been criticized frequently for their tendency to focus on assessing knowledge of isolated facts, thus trivializing what is being tested. Clinical performance-based tests are not immune from similar criticisms. Trivialization in checklist development and in the selection of scoring elements (e.g. in OSCEs) is a danger (Norman, 1990). Unfortunately, it is all too easy to produce a technically reliable test on which the student has been scored on a series of clearly defined criteria that do not reflect the student's real ability or overall performance. The criteria may reflect only those behaviours or skills that are easy to measure while ignoring components of clinical competence that most would agree are more critical and would contribute much more to the validity of the assessment (Norman *et al.*, 1991; van der Vleuten *et al.*, 1991).

Standard setting

Standard setting is the process of determining the score needed to pass an examination (see also Chapters 9 and 15). The true nature of standard setting is often not fully appreciated by medical faculties. This difficulty is due to a lack of understanding that all standard-setting procedures are, to a degree, arbitrary but need not be capricious.

Standard-setting methods are classified commonly as either relative or absolute (Livingston & Zieky, 1982). Relative standards depend on the performance of the examinees taking the examination and are by far the most frequently used. For example, a test in which the lowest scoring 20% of examinees fail, or one in which any examinee scoring less than one standard deviation below the mean fails, has a relative standard.

Absolute standards can be based on an analysis of the content of the examination or by choosing an arbitrary percentage correct for passing; they are independent of the performance of the examinees. Two content-based methods for setting absolute standards on written tests are the Angoff method and the Ebel method (see Chapter 9). Both require a group of experts to review the items or elements on the examination very carefully and to estimate how often a borderline examinee will perform satisfactorily on the item. The Hofstee method is a compromise between absolute and relative standard setting (see Chapter 15).

There is only limited research on standard setting in relation to performance-based tests (Meskauskas, 1986). However, it is our view that, in principle, absolute standards should be used, because whether an examinee passes any given examination should not depend on the performance of other examinees sitting for the examination. Also, we advocate that prior testing results for the elements or items, if they exist, be made available to the judges who set the standards. In addition, consideration should be given to differentiating material into essential and non-essential categories, with different levels required for each.

Reporting scores

Reporting scores is sometimes an area of heated debate (Nungester *et al.*, 1990). In principle, the recipients of the scores and the scale on which they are reported depend on the purpose of the test. It may be that not all recipients should receive the same level of score detail. Regardless of the detail reported, all recipients should receive clearly written material to guide their interpretation of the score information.

Our comments have focused on an examination for graduating medical students and, within this context, it would appear that there are four legitimate recipients of score information. First, one or more persons within the medical school itself need to receive information in order to know whether or not to allow the student to graduate. In some institutions, the recipient is the dean or another administrator; in others, it is a faculty committee. It may be argued that only a pass/fail score is required by the medical school.

Second, the student should receive his or her score. Technically, passing students need receive only a pass/fail score, while failing students need feedback to permit them to assess their strengths and weaknesses. However, it may not be politically acceptable to provide different levels of score specificity to students, and it may be desirable to provide all students with feedback, regardless of their scores on the test. The feedback should be as detailed as possible, within the psychometric and security constraints of the examination.

The third recipient is the institution responsible for keeping records on licensure/credentialing of physicians. Depending on the location, this may be the medical school itself or a local, regional or national agency. A pass/fail score is required.

Finally, teaching faculty need feedback on the performance of the examinees. However, the feedback need not be given in the form of individual scores. It is sufficient to provide teachers with descriptive measures of performance, such as the mean and standard deviation of scores, a frequency distribution of the percentage of cases passed, or other similar anonymous information.

There may be additional issues with tests for other purposes and there may be other legitimate recipients of the test scores. A foremost principle, however, is to avoid the misuse of scores as much as possible. Misuse can be decreased by providing interpretative material with the scores. There is sometimes a tendency, however, for scores to be used for purposes other than the ones for which they were designed, and it is difficult to prevent misuse, short of constraining the dissemination of the information.

Item banking

The term 'item banking' refers to the storage and retrieval of a broad range of testing information. Depending upon the purpose of the bank, it may include the text of the item, information on the item's content, performance information from previous use, and test administration information. Although item banks have been used typically for written items, especially multiple-choice items, they may be developed for other testing modalities as well (e.g. OSCE stations, key-issue simulations).

Reasons for using item banks

Item banking is a powerful tool in the test development, since the accumulation of such information provides a basis for developing tests tailored for a variety of purposes. Each test administration supplies new information that can be stored and used for later test development. Further, item banks can be shared within and across institutions. They may be used to construct complete examinations, to adapt tests to the needs of individual examinees, and to conduct educational research. Modern computer technology makes item banking a viable technique to improve the practice of educational testing (Wood & Skurnik, 1979).

In any education programme, developing and using tests is a time-consuming and difficult task. With item banking, test material can easily be reused and shared, potentially resulting in enormous savings of time and money in the development of new tests. Test designers can review items from the bank systematically, using statistical information about examinee performance to improve item content and phrasing. Over time, as the number of good items increases and poor items are eliminated, the quality of tests as a whole increases.

Computer-based testing

Item banks are typically computer-based, although 'pencil-and-paper' banks are also possible and useful. With additional programming, computers can also be used for interactive test administration, particularly advantageous if instruction is individualized. If appropriate psychometric information has been stored in the bank, adaptive tests can be designed (Wilcox, 1983; Weiss, 1985).

Storage space and, assuming tests are to be scored as well, speed of computation are the key factors in planning for item banks. For most medical school item banks, microcomputers are sufficiently fast, as long as they have a hard disk for data storage. For very large testing programmes (thousands of items and examinees), a minicomputer system may be more desirable.

Meeting software needs is more difficult. It is quite possible, with some programming work, to assemble a workable item banking system from microcomputer-based word processing, database and statistical packages. Alternatively, several integrated item banking systems are available commercially, some with components for computer-based testing, and these should work well for traditional examinations consisting of multiple-choice items.

The pieces of information that should be stored in an item bank depend on the format of the examination used, the specific educational context, and the skills and aspirations of designers and users. For traditional written tests, the bank will store the item text and any associated pictorial information (which may be in separate, hard-copy files). For OSCE-type tests, a broader range of material may be stored, such as a detailed description of the problems, supplemental written test material, special instructions for standardized patients, videotapes of standardized patients for use in training, and scoring information (e.g. checklists, rating forms, answer keys).

Generally, items (or cases) will be classified along a number of dimensions. These may be highly tailored to the specific characteristics of the testing programme (basic science, clinical discipline, examinee task, standardized patient age/sex/race, etc.) or based on taxonomies developed by others. Key words describing item content may also be specified.

Usually item statistics are stored on a computer, the format depending upon the item type. For traditional written test items, indices of item difficulty and discrimination and the distribution of examinee responses would be included typically. For OSCE-type tests, much more information would be stored as well.

Problems encountered in item banking

Although the idea of item banking is simple, and modern equipment is becoming rapidly less expensive, some common problems are encountered during the development of an item bank. Designing a classification system can be a difficult process. If the system is too complex, item classification will be very time consuming. If the system is too simple, the resulting tests may not meet content specifications. Thus, the main purpose of the bank must be clear at the outset, and this should guide the design of the classification system.

Once an item bank is implemented, it is all too easy to add items to the bank and to construct tests from the bank, without careful review. Test quality depends upon systematic review of items.

Computer systems, particularly microcomputer systems, are difficult to protect from unauthorized use. For high-stakes testing, access to the bank must be controlled, both physically and electronically. Files can be password protected and bank contents can be encrypted to reduce the risk of unauthorized access.

Summary

The purpose of this chapter has been to provide a rationale and some guidelines for the development of tests that assess clinical competence. As an example to illustrate some of the topics, we have chosen a test of clinical competence for medical students prior to graduation from medical school. Most of the illustrations have focused on the assessment of skills in patient care, but many of the points we have made are relevant to testing a student's skill in dealing with public health or community-related issues as well.

The comments in this chapter do not represent a complete review of the literature, but, rather, focus on those developments in the testing field, many of them quite recent, that have as a goal the testing of competence in as close to a real-life environment as is feasible. However, it is important to remind ourselves that a comprehensive examination of a graduating student is likely also to include the assessment of subject or disciplinary knowledge and may, quite appropriately, use a variety of testing formats. The point we wish to emphasize is the importance of testing more than the content knowledge assessed typically by written examinations.

The cornerstone of developing a test of clinical competence is careful and thorough planning – identifying the problems, specifying the clinical tasks pertinent to the problems, and preparing a blueprint for the test. Problems that are important should be represented heavily in the blueprint, and should form a large component of the examination. Once these initial planning steps are completed, the test methods that provide the most real-life testing of the problems should be selected for the assessment procedure. Some clinical tasks, such as history taking and communication with the patient, are best assessed in multiple-station (OSCE-type) examinations using standardized patients. There is considerable experience in the effective administration of this examination format, especially in a single site, such as a medical school. Many of the problems related to wide-scale, multi-site testing are being addressed currently by testing agencies in both the USA (the Educational Commission for

Foreign Medical Graduates, the National Board of Medical Examiners) and Canada (the Medical Council of Canada).

Throughout this chapter, a recurring theme was the need for more research, especially in the general areas of scoring and standard setting. A number of specific areas needing additional research have been indicated in our comments. Additionally, comprehensive reviews of the literature, perhaps including a quantitative meta-analysis of unpublished as well as published studies, would be very useful.

Our goal has been to provide some motivation, as well as guidelines, for the development of tests that assess clinical competence. We hope our comments stimulate educators and testing agencies who are pondering the need for such tests to proceed with their development, and encourage those who are involved actively to continue to coordinate their efforts so that their experiences and insights may be shared.

References

American Education Research Association, American Psychological Association and National Council on Measurement in Education (1985). *Standards for Educational and Psychological Testing*. Washington: American Psychological Association.

Barrows, H. S., Neufeld, V. R., Feightner, J. W. & Norman, G. R. (1978). *An Analysis of the Clinical Methods of Medical Students and Physicians*. Toronto: Final Report to Ontario Ministry of Health.

Bordage, G. & Page, G. (1987). An alternative approach to PMPs: the 'key features' concept. In *Further Developments in Assessing Clinical Competence*, ed. I. R. Hart & R. M. Harden, pp. 59–72. Montreal: Can-Heal Publications.

Cole, N. S. & Moss, P. A. (1989). Bias in test use. In *Educational Measurement*, 3rd edn, ed. R. L. Linn, pp. 201–19. New York: MacMillan.

Colliver, J. A., Verhulst, S. J., Williams, R. G. & Norcini, J. J. (1989). Reliability of performance on standardized patient cases: a comparison of consistency measures based on generalisability theory. *Teaching and Learning in Medicine*, **1**, 31–7.

Colliver, J. A., Vu, N. V. & Barrows, H. S. (1992). Screening test length and pass–fail cut-offs for sequential testing with a standardized-patient based examination: a receiver operating characteristic (ROC) analysis. *Academic Medicine*, **67**, 592–5.

Ebel, R. L. (1983). The practical validation of tests of ability. *Educational Measurement: Issues and Practice*, **2**, 7–10.

Elstein, A., Shulman, L. & Sprafka, S. (1978). *Medical Problem Solving*. Cambridge: Harvard University Press.

Frederiksen, N. (1984). The real test bias. *American Psychologist*, **37**, 911–18.

Kane, M. T. (1982). The validity of licensure examinations. *American Psychologist*, **37**, 911–18.

Livingston, S. A. & Zieky, M. J. (1982). *Passing Scores*. Princeton: Educational Testing Service.

Meskauskas, J. A. (1986). Setting standards for credentialing examinations. *Evaluation in the Health Professions*, **9**, 187–203.

Neufeld, V. R. & Norman, G. R. (Eds.) (1985). *Assessing Clinical Competence*. New York: Springer.

Newble, D. I. (1992). Assessing clinical competence at the undergraduate level. ASME Medical Education Booklet Number 25. *Medical Education*, **26**, 504–11.

Newble, D. I. & Jaeger, K. (1983). The effect of assessments and examinations on the learning of medical students. *Medical Education*, **17**, 165–71.

Newble, D. I. & Swanson, D. B. (1988) Psychometric characteristics of the objective structured clinical examination. *Medical Education*, **22**, 325–34.

Norcini, J. J., Swanson, D. B., Webster, G. D. & Grosso, L. J. (1983). A comparison of several methods for scoring patient management problems. *Proceedings of the 22nd Annual Conference on Research in Medical Education*, pp. 41–6. Washington: Association of American Medical Colleges.

Norman, G. R. (1988). Problem-solving skills, solving problems and problem-based learning. *Medical Education*, **22**, 279–86.

Norman, G. R. (1990). Summary of the conference. In *Teaching and Assessing Clinical Competence*, ed. W. Bender, R. J. Heimstra, A. J. J. A. Scherpbier & R. P. Zwierstra, pp. 599–609. Groningen: BoekWerk Publications.

Norman, G. R., van der Vleuten, C. P. M. & de Graaff, E. (1991). Pitfalls in the pursuit of objectivity: issues of validity, efficiency and acceptability. *Medical Education*, **25**, 119–26.

Nungester, R. J., Dawson-Saunders, B., Kelley, P. R. & Volle, R. L. (1990). Score reporting on NBME examinations. *Academic Medicine*, **12**, 723–9.

Peterson, N. S., Kolen, M. J. & Hoover, H. D. (1989). Scaling, norming and equating. In *Educational Measurement*, 3rd edn, ed. R. L. Linn, pp. 221–62. New York: MacMillan.

Rothman, A. I., Cohen, R., Dawson-Saunders, B., Poldre, P. P. & Ross, J. (1992). Testing the equivalence of multiple-station tests of clinical competence. *Academic Medicine*, **67**, 40–1.

Rutala, P. J., Witzke, D. B. & Fulginiti, J. V. (1991). The influence of student and standardized patient gender on scoring in an objective structured clinical examination. *Academic Medicine*, **66**, S28–S30.

Skaggs, G. & Lissitz, R. W. (1986). IRT test equating: relevant issues and a review of recent research. *Review of Educational Research*, **56**, 495–529.

Swanson, D. B. (1987). A measurement framework for performance-based tests. In *Further Developments in Assessing Clinical Competence*, ed. I. R. Hart & R. M. Harden, pp. 13–45. Montreal: Can-Heal Publications.

Swanson, D. B. & Norcini, J. J. (1989). Factors influencing the reproducibility of tests using standardized patients. *Teaching and Learning in Medicine*, **1**, 158–66.

Swanson, D. B., Norcini, J. J. & Grosso, L. J. (1987). Assessment of clinical competence: written and computer-based simulations. *Assessment and Evaluation in Higher Education*, **12**, 220–46.

Tamblyn, R. (1989). 'Use of Standardized Patients in the Assessment of Clinical Competence'. Ph.D. Dissertation, Montreal: McGill University.

Tamblyn, R. M., Klass, D. J., Schnable, G. K. & Kopelow, M. L. (1991). Sources of unreliability and bias in standardized-patient ratings. *Teaching and Learning in Medicine*, **3**, 74–85.

van der Vleuten, C. P. M. & Swanson, D. B. (1990). Assessment of clinical skills with standardised patients: state of the art. *Teaching and Learning in Medicine*, **2**, 58–76.

van der Vleuten, C. P. M., Norman, G. R. & de Graaff, E. (1991). Pitfalls in the pursuit of objectivity: issues of reliability. *Medical Education*, **25**, 110–18.

Wakeford, R. E. (Ed.) (1985) *Directions in Clinical Assessment*. Proceedings of the First Cambridge Conference. Cambridge: Cambridge University School of Medicine.

Weiss, D. J. (1985). Adaptive testing by computer. *Journal of Consulting and Clinical Psychology*, **53**, 774–89.

Wilcox, R. R. (1983). Unbiased estimation in a closed sequential testing procedure. *Educational and Psychological Measurement*, **43**, 1061–3.

Wood, R. & Skurnik, L. S. (1979). *Item banking: a method for producing school-based examinations and nationally comparable grades*. National Foundation for Educational Research in England and Wales.

7

Determining the content of certifying examinations

DALE DAUPHINEE (Editor), WESLEY FABB,
BRIAN JOLLY, DONALD LANGSLEY,
STEPHEN WEALTHALL and PETER PROCOPIS

The content of any certifying or evaluation process, be it one examination or a series of evaluating instruments, must be based on a definition of what is expected of the candidates. There are several reasons why a precise definition of content must be determined before the specific tests or measuring methods are developed. The first is that it must be absolutely clear to candidates and examiners what knowledge, skills, behavior or attitudes are expected and will be evaluated. A general definition of content is not sufficient, for example, 'the skills and knowledge necessary for a general internist in a small North American town' is not helpful. While this would be a good starting point, a more precise identification is needed to help to guarantee a more reliable and valid examination. When both examiners and candidates know the potential content of the tests, candidates can be better prepared and, equally important for the candidates, the examiners and test builders will reflect the same content in the examination. Another reason for the precise definition of content is the need for fairness and the appearance of fairness in the legal sense. Currently, North American courts have become interested in the job relatedness of tests and evaluation. If an examination is arbitary and not job related, the unsuccessful candidate has a strong basis to initiate an appeal. A final reason is that the public expects the process of certification, be it for licensure, registration or specialty certificate, to assess those attributes which it expects the practitioner to demonstrate in day-to-day practice. Increasing participation by the public in professional bodies is a reflection of this concern. These reasons are magnified when one begins to tackle the issue of recertification where content varies considerably from one setting to another and assessment must focus on actual practice. For a more detailed discussion of these issues, the reader is referred to Neufeld (1985a), Rogers (1988), Langsley (1991) and Chapter 13.

Model

The general model to be followed in this discussion is that laid out by Newble *et al.* in Chapter 6. Since the focus of this discussion will be on knowledge as related to performance 'on the job' and performance assessment (doing, not just knowing how to do), this particular approach is very appropriate. For an excellent overview of these distinctions, the review by Miller is recommended (Miller, 1990). Similarly, because the certification target is oriented usually towards patient-related skills and knowledge, one can view the identification of the content for any certification process in the same way that one thinks of sampling in an epidemiological or clinical study. First the target population of patients is identified, then a representative sample of individuals is drawn from it. Thus, the point of the exercise is to develop a process whereby, firstly, one determines the specific clinical role for which one wants to certify the candidate, secondly, one determines the knowledge, skills and attitudes which are specific to that role (the role content), and finally one determines the examination blueprint and sampling process whereby one selects those items, stations, etc. for the actual test which candidates will receive (the examination content). Our task in this paper is to expand on this approach by determining the clinical setting (role and content) to which one wishes to generalize and then by setting the examination's content to reflect that target.

Factors influencing content decisions

Having reviewed the general approach and model underlying this discussion and having discussed the concept of content, there are several factors which must be considered in making decisions about content. These factors influence the content decisions but do not alter the basic model. They could be thought of as a checklist of issues to be considered in order to ensure that the evaluation fits the intended role more specifically and more efficiently.

Stage of training and experience

The importance of the target candidates' experience or stage of training is an obvious concern in designing the evaluation. However, it is being suggested that in certification the focus should not be on what the candidate has done but rather on the stage to which the candidate is moving. For instance, the focus for a senior medical student, might be the role of a trainee intern, or, if a senior resident physician, the focus might be on the expected demands of independent practice which will be encountered in the foreseeable future. Generally speaking, there are four typical levels where certification (in a generic sense) is utilized: entry into postgraduate training after medical school; entry into general licensure; entry into specialty practice (this can be of a good general orientation as in family medicine certification in North America or very specialized as in the case of pediatric cardiology) and recertification. The latter presents a very specific challenge and will be considered in Part D.

National (or regional) model of licensure

How does the licensure model make an impact on the evaluation process? This is not an obvious question. One might ask whether it matters if the specific model of licensure grants a general license or defines two tracks of licensure, such as family medicine and specialty practice. Let one suppose that we wish to certify a general internist and that the local licensure model provides for general licensure with a common entry examination for all forms of practice. Then the certification evaluation for internists can be more focused. In the reverse situation, one may wish to insert an evaluation bias in the entry to specialty examination to cover the eventualities of the general licensure model. On the other hand, there may be problems with omissions in the licensure examination, and one still has the opportunity to 'cover' those aspects in the certification process. These scenarios illustrate exactly why content must be specified in advance.

Style of practice

The impact of the style of practice applies to licensure and certification but even more so to recertification and the subsequent stages of the continuum of clinical evaluation. The examining body, which is responsible for the examination, may wish to introduce elements to assess rural versus urban practice differentially, or special interest skills within the various specialty certificates (e.g. ultrasound skills within the cardiologist certificate). Two special situations to be considered are the requirements for unusual practice environments such as very remote practice sites like northern Canada or the Australian outback and, at the other extreme, the academic role. In the latter case, special skills are monitored usually by the peer review process of the university. However, unusual preparation or background for the academic physicians who have trained in another jurisdiction may require a site-specific evaluation (e.g. knowledge of specific public health laws, etc.).

The dangerous physician

Many expect that certifying, and particularly recertifying, systems will pick up the dangerous practitioner. They may, but such systems should not be expected to do so unless specific elements of content and, most importantly, scoring are designed to achieve that purpose (Mankin, 1987; Kramer, 1990). If there is perception of a problem with dangerous practitioners, generally speaking, more specific instruments (tests, evaluations, etc.) or processes should be designed to meet that purpose. For example, dangerous behavior on the part of an anesthetist in hospital is best dealt with by quality assurance programmes at the hospital in the latter case, and by recertifying procedures in the case of the outdated internist.

Values and accountability

There is growing concern that many groups perceive the medical profession as lacking in humanistic values and a sense of accountability to the public (Association of American Medical Colleges, 1984). Similarly, there is a perceived need to emphasize values, be they related to ethical issues or the acknowledgement that cultural values of patients influence attitudes to illness and health, and that practitioners must be trained and prepared to deal with such issues (Pellegrino, 1989). Thus, in determining content, one must make a conscious decision to define such content, which will vary from country to country, and of course to determine how it will be evaluated. It is probably fair to state that content pertaining to values can no longer be evaluated or defined as a generic category like 'ethical behavior or ethics' on an in-training report. It must be explicitly defined and evaluated in each practice environment for each certification process (see Chapter 13).

Very much at the heart of these perceptions is the notion of the accountability of the profession which must be acknowledged and defined for each certification procedure. Accountability includes responsibilities to patients and their families, to the community and to the public at large through regulating bodies such as licensing and certifying bodies.

Technical issues

A series of technical, fiscal and legal issues also confront the decision maker when defining content. Some authors refer to these as issues of feasibility (Neufeld, 1985*b*). They deal with the practical questions of what is possible and practical as opposed to the ideal!

Resources

What can the sponsoring organization afford to do? How much money does it have to spend? What kind of human resources are available to deal with not only technical issues like psychometric properties of tests, but also the practical issues of supervizing examination sites and maintaining question banks (see Chapters 6, 8 and 9)? Often some resources, such as technical supports, can be shared with similar organizations.

Limitation of instruments

In this instance, we are referring to both written and practical-based 'instruments' like multiple-choice examinations, in-training reports and objective structured clinical examinations (OSCEs). Can the existing instruments measure what is being asked or will new ones be needed? Can the proposed instruments measure what is being asked in a reasonable length of time and still be reliable? In this instance, technical help is needed early on in determining content, so that measurement problems are anticipated, and all alternatives are considered in advance of final decisions about evaluation models (Neufeld, 1985*b*).

Legal issues

While not the initial concern of content, the notions of following principles of natural justice and not discriminating against individuals must be kept in mind (O'Brien, 1986; Irby & Milan, 1989). Similarly, potential legal challenges based on shortcomings of the proposed instruments must be considered in the planning stages.

Special challenges

Research in the areas of psychology and educational measurement has presented two issues which have provided particular challenges to the test developers.

Cognitive models

Over the last 10 years, clinical problem-solving and decision-making has been shown to differ between novices, those with intermediate experience and experts. Furthermore, even within groups of experts, different approaches are used depending on the degree of expertise, knowledge and experience (Norman, 1989). This alerts one to the possibility that examination-induced reasoning artefacts may occur if the examination is not cognitively sound. To be even more provocative, does one design questions at the expert level only or does one design them at an intermediate or sub-expert level, for example, when examining candidates at the mid-training level? The question has not been answered but it is probably safe to say that questions which are focused on the process of reasoning (e.g. what question would you ask the patient next) versus the outcome (e.g. what is the diagnosis) must be created with care and emphasis should be placed on 'outcome' measures, studies have shown that experts may use several approaches and different content to solve a problem (Patel & Groen, 1991). Again, expert advice is indicated once one has reached that stage of test development.

Content specificity

A second issue, related to the previous topic, is content specificity. Given the variation in experience and expertise, to what extent does one sample each content area? To rephrase the question, it is clear that knowledge and experience are needed to develop expertise, yet we know student and professional experience and expertise varies considerably from situation to situation (van der Vleuten & Norman, 1991). Therefore, to what extent does one test each area of expertise? For example, for a graduating student, does one sample by traditional topics like medicine and pediatrics or by other broad areas like emergency, prevention, etc. until one can get a reliable score, or does one look at subsets like emergency-elderly? There is no clear answer but again an empirical decision can be made with expert advice.

Steps to determine content

As noted previously, the general approach which is being suggested follows the model described in Chapter 6. That approach defined three steps to be followed, discussed below.

Step 1: Identify the clinical problems the student should be able to handle to some degree of resolution

Since emphasis is being placed on assessment of actual performance, the test developer should define content by means of problems which will present in real life to the practitioners or trainees being assessed. For example, for an individual dealing with a geriatric population, a presenting problem could be the disoriented patient or, for a general practitioner, acute abdominal pain in a middle-aged man.

The focus at this step is to define presenting clinical problems. The defining of specific skills and tasks involved in dealing with the presenting problem is Step 2. A classification of presenting problems is recommended strongly. For example, one may define the population by age group on one axis, by body system on another and by acuity and impact on a third axis. While a classification is not a crucial decision in Step 1, it is most helpful when a sampling strategy is established in Step 3, and must be completely compatible with the eventual examination sampling grid. That will be discussed in more detail later.

A major component in defining the presenting problems is actually how to identify valid clinical problems (Linn, 1984). Preferably, this is done from existing data (practice profiles) or observation in actual practice settings. Furthermore, the problems must be site and target-group specific. For example, a practice profile for a rural general practitioner in the American West is of some help and relevance but is incomplete in assessing an internist in a teaching hospital in Australia or for a graduating student in New Zealand.

Obviously, this exercise is not usually done from scratch for each site owing to cost considerations. Fortunately, several sources can be considered, which are discussed below.

Encounter sheets or practice logs

These sources often use presenting complaints or problems, rather than diagnosis, and are most useful if valid. For example, for definition of training programmes for nurses in northern Canada, logs from nursing stations were most helpful in identifying presenting problems for their curriculum and their evaluation (Dauphinee, 1970).

Data banks

Often the data banks of third-party payers or other insuring bodies may provide a definition of presenting problems. Unfortunately, such banks often deal in diagnosis rather than presenting problems, which may limit their usefulness in identifying patients' modes of presentation.

Surveys of physicians

Some organizations survey their members or a sample of their membership and these can be a source of problems (Langsley & Hollender, 1982; Langsley & Yager, 1988). The principal problem with this source is the validity of the data elicited: is it data by recall or actual review of practice records? Objective sources of data are preferable as recall of practice content may be unreliable (Curry & Putnam, 1981).

Creating 'hypothetical profiles'

An interesting approach is to take data from several sources and to create a series of problems using a hypothetical physician's practice profile. This approach has been used by both American and Canadian groups. The approach requires experts' judgements, perhaps using consensus generating techniques like the Delphi method.

Miscellaneous 'indirect' data sources

In keeping with the previous option, several sources of data can contribute to developing a profile of problems (Norman, 1985). They include epidemiological or demographic data that can establish age profiles or the incidence of certain chronic diseases for the practice location under consideration. Similarly, the nature of health resources and specific health issues of concern in a specific community (e.g. the disabled or an inner city population) may also influence the selection of problems for an assessment exercise. Thus, the gathering of data from consumers is important and adds greatly to the face validity of the evaluation. A variation on this theme is to prime the target group under evaluation with respect to a new medical development which may represent either a new problem or, as it is often the case, a new therapy. In either case, these various sources of data or consumer opinion are especially useful in creating problems for 'a hypothetical practice'.

Step 2: For each problem, define the clinical tasks in which the examinee is expected to be competent

This step is basically the exercise of identifying the tasks or actions specific for each presenting problem. The traditional approach of defining tasks and actions is considered too limited by today's standards because of new methods of evaluation which allow one to explore a wider range of tasks (Miller, 1990).

Examples of new developments would be the use of standardized patients to address issues in the clinical interview or the OSCE to assess communication skills such as the handling of an anxious parent on the phone. A list of non-traditional tasks to be considered is:

(i) The responsiveness of the practitioner to the patient, to society, to self and family and the sensitivity to ethical issues
(ii) Aspects of communication which emphasize non-diagnostic related skills such as patient comprehension and compliance
(iii) Familiarity with issues of resource (human and fiscal) allocation including support structures (family, community, self-help groups, etc.)
(iv) Methods of quality assurance relevant to clinical practice: not just those in a hospital context
(v) The efficient use of resources
(vi) Self-directed development in order to cope better with the changing nature of practice and the medical and social sciences and including notions of self-audit and critical appraisal

Obviously, the so-called classical or conventional actions and tasks of the clinician are still very important. These actions include: the history and the physical examination; the investigation of problems by laboratory methods and diagnostic procedures; the treatment and management options; the prevention strategies; and perhaps, most importantly, the interpretation and participant communication of the results to the patient, the family and the rest of the health team.

In conclusion, the purpose of this step is to assign actions and tasks specific to each presenting clinical problem. The point of emphasis is to think beyond the usual and time-limited tasks and skills which have consumed our attention as clinical evaluators over the years. These newer tasks should focus on responsiveness, non-diagnostic related communication, self-directed development, efficiency and smart allocation and utilization of human and fiscal resources by the physician of the 1990s. In each examination instance, this list of established and innovative actions must be adopted for the level of training and stage of development for each target group.

Step 3: Prepare a blue-print to guide in the selection of problems to be included in the assessment procedure

At this juncture, one has a series of presenting problems and the appropriate clinical tasks specific for each problem. Now one is faced with the chore of developing a taxonomy or classification of problems and tasks with which to build the evaluation or examination. An analogy might be the building of a library: first, one decides on broad categories of books or software (i.e. presenting problems) like clinical medicine, health and epidemiology which represent the broad educational goals of the institution (i.e. practice location). Next, the specific topics or titles (i.e. actions or tasks) for each category are considered for each level of education (i.e. undergraduate, postgraduate). Having compiled these lists, one uses a classification system (e.g. national library index) around which one files and organizes the material. This is followed by developing a process with which the actual selection of books and software is made (selecting a sample) for each purpose given learning method and resources. Without forcing the analogy, in our present task, one now has reached the step of classification: selecting the content and developing the questions and/or stations to meet each objective. This, in turn, is followed by another Step, which can be done only after Steps 1–3 are accomplished. That is the selection of test methods (see Chapters 6 and 8).

Newble *et al.* give a succinct summary about the issue of the use of blueprints (see Chapter 6). Essentially, test blueprints or question grids for specific examinations can be simple or complex. Several factors may influence how many axes or dimensions are essential to the design. To start, the dimensions of the selected blueprint should reflect a valid balancing of health care goals as well as the needs of the population to be served. For general licensure, the axes might be age, prevalence and health impact. For a consulting specialty, the axes might be prevalence, type of consultative role (e.g. diagnostic or therapeutic problem) and body system. Secondly, while computers allow multi-dimensional modeling, it is probably advisable to keep any blueprint on question grid limited to three dimensions. Thirdly, preparing a blueprint, because it is best limited to three dimensions, requires that test makers be sensitive that other aspects of clinical activity independent of the blueprint content are represented appropriately across individual items: neither too few manual tasks or an excessive number of therapeutic acts across all situations.

There are two consequences to this step: a blueprint is developed to select an appropriate sample of problems and tasks which accurately represent the reality of the practice setting to which one wishes to generalize the results (recall the analogy of epidemiology and how the sample of people must represent the population to which one wishes to generalize) and also allows one to design the bank of problems, cases or other examination components to meet the measurement needs. To illustrate this latter point, one has the means to classify the bank of examination questions or stations and to find the holes (e.g. there are no questions to deal with prevention in heart disease) and to develop the missing components. Thus, the blueprint is a method of setting a valid examination and also validating the content of the examination bank.

To summarize, the blueprint is not only a means to have a valid list or bank of questions and problems, but also a valid examination which reflects the component skills and the exact context and situation in which the task is executed. Thereby, one guarantees that tasks are tested, not as isolated acts (e.g. examine the seventh cranial nerve), but as acts in the context of a presenting problem (e.g. given a history compatible with a Bell's palsy, how does the candidate assess the problem, including examining the seventh cranial nerve).

Before concluding the discussion on blueprints, a series of subpoints must be made.

(i) The introduction of testing over a period of time may be a possibility. For example, certification may be a series of steps over two or three years or, in recertification, may proceed over a lifetime! This does not change the basic process but allows one merely to cover more material and more situations, if needed, than in a 'one shot'

(ii) The concept of testing over time may not be simply complementary but actually sequential. For example, one could use common or typical problems in the early stages and the less common and more atypical ones as expertise develops in later stages of assessment. This is a means of taking a clinical task and expanding the role over time

(iii) In an examination, there may be a desire to consider certain tasks as essential and therefore these must be answered correctly. This is a reasonable approach but has major consequences for scoring and standard setting (see Chapters 9 and 10). This, again, will require expert advice and planning in advance

Summary

This overview has been directed towards medical practitioners or other health professionals who find themselves thrust into the certification or licensure process without the benefit of previous training or preparation. We have tried to describe an approach for building examinations and evaluations which aims to be as fair and as valid as possible and therefore legally defensible. We have built on the model of Newble *et al.* (see Chapter 6) into which some of us had input because it is workable, up-to-date and field tested. Similarly, certifying organizations contemplating change will find this material of use in preparing their examination committees. However used, we would emphasize the crucial need to have a process which is valid and job related and an examination structure which will contribute ultimately to the improvement of examination reliability.

References

Association of American Medical Colleges (1984). *Panel on the General Professional Education of the Physician and College Preparation for Medicine. Physicians for the Twenty-First Century: The GPEP Report.* Washington: Association of American Medical Colleges.

Curry, L. & Putnam, R. W. (1981). Accuracy of physicians' self-reported practice profiles. *Proceedings of Twentieth Annual Conference of Research in Medical Education*, pp. 29–33. Washington: Association of American Medical Colleges.

Dauphinee, W. D. (1970). *Report on Clinical Training of Nurses for Medical Services in the North*. Department of National Health and Welfare, Canada.

Irby, D. M. & Milan, S. (1989). The legal context for evaluating and dismissing medical students and residents. *Academic Medicine*, **54**, 639–43.

Kramer, B. A. (1990). A follow-up study of 'dangerous answers' in four medical specialties. *Evaluation in the Health Professions*, **13**, 489–503.

Langsley, D. G. (1991). Medical competence and performance assessment: a new era. *Journal of American Medical Association*, **266**, 977–80.

Langsley, D. G. & Hollender, M. H. (1982). The definition of a psychiatrist. *American Journal of Psychiatry*, **139**, 81–5.

Langsley, D. G. & Yager, J. (1988). The definition of a psychiatrist: eight years later. *American Journal of Psychiatry*, **145**, 469–75.

Linn, R. C. (1984). Standards for validity in licensure testing. *Professions Education Researcher Notes*, **6**, 13–4.

Mankin, H. (1987). Pilot study using 'dangerous answers' as a scoring technique on certifying exams. *Journal of Medical Education*, **62**, 621–4.

Miller, G. E. (1990). The assessment of clinical skills, competence, performance. *Academic Medicine*, **65**, 563–7.

Neufeld, V. R. (1985*a*). Historical perspective on clinical competence. In *Assessing Clinical Competence*, ed. V. R. Neufeld & G. R. Norman, pp. 3–14. New York: Springer Publishing Company.

Neufeld, V. R. (1985*b*). An introduction to measurement properties. In *Assessing Clinical Competence*, ed. V. R. Neufeld & G. R. Norman, pp. 39–50. New York: Springer Publishing Company.

Norman, G. R. (1985). Defining competence: a methodological review. In *Assessing Clinical Competence*, ed. V. R. Neufeld & G. R. Norman, pp. 15–35. New York: Springer Publishing Company.

Norman, G. R. (Ed.) (1989). 'The psychology of clinical reasoning: implications for assessment'. Paper from the Fourth Cambridge Conference on Medical Education. Cambridge, 5–11 June, 1989.

O'Brien, T. L. (1986). Legal trends affecting the validity of credentialing examinations. *Evaluation and the Health Professions*, **9**, 171–85.

Patel, V. & Groen, G. J. (1991). The general and specific nature of medical expertise: a critical look. In *Toward a General Theory of Expertise, Properties and Limits*, ed. K. A. Ericsson & J. Smith, pp. 93–125. Cambridge: Cambridge University Press.

Pellegrino, E. D. (1989). Teaching medical ethics: some persistent questions and some responses. *Academic Medicine*, **64**, 701–3.

Rogers, D. E. (1988). Clinical education and the doctor of tomorrow. In *Adopting Clinical Medical Education to the Needs of Today and Tomorrow*, ed. B. Gastel & D. E. Rogers. New York: The New York Academy of Medicine.

van der Vleuten, C. & Norman, G. R. (1991). 'Implications of research on licensure and certification for recertification'. Position Paper for Cambridge Conference, University of Adelaide 1991.

8

Methods of assessment in certification

CEES van der VLEUTEN and DAVID NEWBLE
(Editors), SUSAN CASE, GARETH HOLSGROVE,
BARRIE McCANN, COLIN McRAE and
NICHOLAS SAUNDERS

The assessment of clinical competence has been characterized by a wealth of test methods each purporting to measure various aspects or components of competence. Many are represented by acronyms (e.g. MCQ, MEQ, PMP, CBX, SP, OSCE; see Figure 8.1) and several useful reference texts are available (e.g. Fabb & Marshall, 1983; Neufeld & Norman, 1985; Wakeford, 1985). Additional methods have been introduced from time to time, usually promising a new solution to an important measurement problem. Often the initial optimism has been tempered subsequently by empirical evidence of the limitations of the new approach. Nevertheless, there has been a gradual improvement in the range and quality of test methods. On the other hand, in the real world of undergraduate education, it is clear that the choice of methods used for the measurement of clinical competence is often governed as much by personal experiences, traditions and 'gut feelings' as by a rational consideration of the published literature on assessment and an understanding of the strengths and weaknesses of the tools at our command.

The main purpose of this chapter is to bring some organization into the selection of methods for the assessment of clinical competence. However, it is not intended as a comprehensive review of all available methods nor will it provide a practical 'how to do it' guide. Rather, a number of methods will be discussed to illustrate major shifts in the evolution of clinical competence assessment. This discussion will be based on the substantial experimental and empirical data which has accumulated in recent years.

A historical perspective

In attempting to provide an overview of methods used for the assessment of clinical competence it is interesting, as well as helpful, to take a

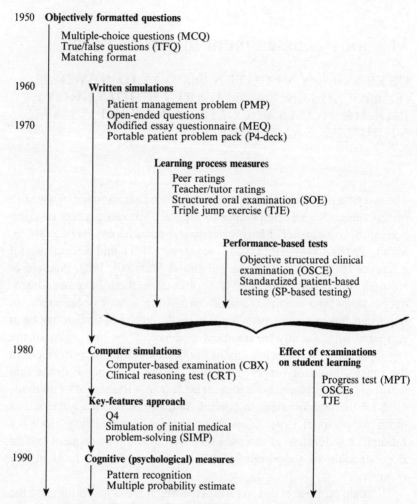

Fig. 8.1. Historical overview of methods used in clinical competence assessment.

historical perspective. A schematic representation is provided in Figure 8.1. It shows a time scale for the major innovations in methodology over the last four decades. Such a representation allows us to map a number of important changes in the assessment of competence and in the types of method which have been developed (the appendix to this Chapter contains a list of general and specific references for the instruments listed in Figure 8.1).

Objective tests

The overview starts in the 1950s, a period where higher education was characterized by a marked increase in student enrolments, a change which included the medical school. From an assessment point of view, the era was notable for the introduction of 'objective' tests (e.g. multiple choice questions (MCQs)). This trend was probably accelerated with the advent of the computer. Today it would be hard to find a medical school or licensing body that is not making extensive use of computer-marked objective-type tests. In many institutions such tests rapidly became the predominant method of assessment, often replacing the traditional essay tests and even viva voce and bedside oral examinations.

As experience with objective-type tests grew, a feeling of dissatisfaction emerged. There was a concern that such tests tended to measure merely rote-learned knowledge and, hence, were an inappropriate approach to the assessment of higher levels of cognitive functioning and of the active application of knowledge. The MCQ format, with its list of options, was thought to provide assistance to the examinee in choosing the correct response (cueing). Thus, the MCQ (and its many variants) was considered by some to be unsuitable for use in tests of clinical competence because of its low fidelity.

Simulations

The dissatisfaction with methods existing in the 1950s led to the development of a multitude of new instruments in the 1960s. The focus of interest became the application of knowledge in the clinical context – or clinical problem-solving. As a general basis, some simulation of reality was used to enhance fidelity. An examinee was confronted with a practical situation, usually a patient-case. The route taken and the decisions made were used to quantify the candidates' problem-solving ability.

The most widely known instrument in this category became known as the patient management problem (PMP). Some PMPs were fairly simple and used a linear development of the problem. Others were more ingenious and allowed various paths of progress through the case (branching PMPs). Ingenious techniques were developed to allow selective disclosure of information and to prevent cueing. Subsequently, computer techniques took over these functions and encouraged even more complexity. In the 1970s, PMPs became very popular and were incorporated into national licensing examinations (e.g. the American

National Boards). In the 1980s high technology has been used to incorporate pictorial images and real-time changes into the simulation (e.g. computer-based examination (CBX)).

In addition to written and computer-based PMPs, other simulation techniques were introduced. One example is the structured oral examination (SOE) in which the examiner plays the role of the patient and assessor concurrently, using a structured protocol for information giving and scoring.

One of the major disadvantages of using simulation as a testing method has been the scoring of examinee performance. As the complexity of simulations increased this became more of a puzzle. Problems included the weighting of choices, the scoring of sequences and the value to be accorded comprehensiveness as opposed to efficiency. A common way of developing scores was to use the opinions or performance of experts but with increasing complexity the less consensus there appeared to be on the appropriateness of actions and answers. Several marking systems have been developed (see Swanson *et al.*, 1987) but scoring problems remain a serious impediment to the use of instruments based on simulation.

In the 1980s it became apparent that there was another major disadvantage associated with simulations. The results of research indicated consistently that performance on one simulation was a very poor predictor of performance on another simulation. This undermined the basis of the developmental philosophy behind simulations: that they were measuring 'problem-solving ability' as a broad attribute and one relatively independent of the problem being simulated. The research now showed that competence at problem-solving was highly dependent on the content of the particular case and a change in case content, sometimes even a minimal change, yielded a totally different performance. Consequently, to achieve a reliable assessment of clinical problem-solving performance many simulations or cases are required. This finding has major implications for simulations in current use, since most are complex and time consuming. Reliability can be achieved only through long testing times, often lasting a day or more.

Improving the efficiency of testing methods has now become an issue for overcoming the problem of content specificity. One of the most creative solutions came from the First Cambridge Conference. It was suggested that instead of working through a complete patient problem chronologically, only those parts of the case be simulated which contained the components critical to the solution of the problem. In any one case the critical area could be within the history taking, the physical examination, the investigation or the management. For testing purposes, it would suffice to target these key components and to skip the other elements of the case without loss of information on the candidates' competence. Originally, these simulations became known as 'Cambridge cases' (Norman *et al.*, 1985) and later as the 'key-features approach' (Bordage & Page, 1987). Relatively few instruments of this type have appeared but examples include the simulation of initial problem solving (SIMP) and the so-called Q4 project of the Medical Council of Canada (Q4 has no particular significance other than indicating the fourth component of the Medical Council's Qualifying Examination). Such instruments commence with a case description which is then followed by MCQ or free-response-type questions.

New concepts of clinical problem-solving

In the 1970s and 1980s several studies showed that expert clinicians often performed little better than less experienced doctors on simulations of clinical problem-solving (Friedman *et al.*, 1978; McLeskey & Ward, 1978; Grant & Marsden, 1988; Schmidt *et al.*, 1990). Initially, this was attributed to technical limitations of the instruments, such as the scoring system. Other concerns were raised when it was shown that performance on simulations correlated very highly with MCQ examinations, indicating that relatively little unique information was gathered by the simulation and it was at high cost (Norcini *et al.*, 1985).

Such studies have challenged afresh those researchers concerned to develop valid tests of clinical problem-solving. Within these paradigms, elegant tests were produced which appeared to represent reality but failed to discriminate between different levels of competency.

The 1990s will see the taking aboard of new theoretical knowledge from cognitive psychological research on the nature of problem-solving and expert-novice differences. (Norman *et al.*, 1990; Schmidt *et al.*, 1990). This chapter on test methods is not the place for a treatise on psychology. However, some information from this area may be of value to test developers. First, problem-solving is not measurable as a consistent trait (like a personality trait). Second, knowledge is important in all stages of expertise but the way it is stored and retrieved changes with growing expertise. Third, expertise develops as a transition from a conceptually rich and rational knowledge base (acquired from educational experiences) to a non-analytical ability to recognize and handle situations efficiently and effectively (acquired from extensive clinical experiences). Thus, at the highest level of functioning, the expert uses a sophisticated form of pattern recognition characterized by speed and efficient use of information.

At this point we are at the cutting edge of test development. Preliminary attempts are being made to transpose the experimental laboratory instruments of the psychologists into practical methods of testing competence (Norman, 1989). Others are attempting to modify current test methods (e.g. MCQs) to take into account these new concepts (Case *et al.*, 1991). It seems certain that, in the future, measurements of competence will include tests of knowledge, but the knowledge will be assessed within very realistic contexts.

Learning process measures

The 1970s saw many innovations in medical education such as problem-based learning. The emphasis by now had shifted from *teaching* to *student learning* and, in line with these developments, attempts were made to assess the learning process used by students.

An example is the triple jump exercise (TJE) which was designed to assess the quality of students' problem-analysis and information-gathering skills. The TJE consists of three steps (jumps): a structured oral based usually on a patient's problem; a time-limited (e.g. 24 hours) study assignment; a repeat structured oral in which the success of the assignment is probed.

Other illustrations of process measures are various forms of self, peer or faculty ratings in which qualities such as the ability to collaborate, task orientedness and communication skills are assessed. However, such instruments have never been introduced on a large scale, mainly due to their poor psychometric qualities (Case *et al.* 1991).

Effect of assessment on student learning

In the 1980s there arose a growing awareness of the enormous influence of examinations on student learning. It seemed that examinations often determined the curriculum rather than vice versa. Examples have been described where assessment procedures were devised with the specific objective of driving learning in a favourable direction. In one such procedure, a new test of clinical competence was developed to balance the observed undesirable effects of the knowledge-based MCQ tests in a final examination (Newble & Jaeger, 1983). The Maastricht progress test (MPT) provides another illustration of this strategy (van der Vleuten & Verwijnen, 1990). The MPT is an MCQ-type test of knowledge which consists of a sample of questions based on the outcome objectives of the curriculum. It is administered periodically to all students irrespective of their year of study. This makes it impossible for students to prepare specifically for the test but individual ongoing study is rewarded by the demonstration of progressive improvement in the knowledge base.

Such studies have demonstrated that examinations are powerful motivating subsystems within the educational environment. Used with care and skill, this understanding provides a way of achieving substantial educational change. To do so in a way which will enhance the success of the curriculum will require a more central and sophisticated approach to assessment than is usual in most medical schools.

Performance-based tests

A concern about the reliability of traditional clinical examinations voiced in the 1960s led to attempts to standardize the conditions under which such examinations were conducted. The development in the 1970s of the objective structured clinical examination (OSCE) (Harden & Gleeson, 1979) and other variants of the multiple-station approach has had an enormous impact. Such performance-based tests often include simulations with high fidelity (e.g. standardized patients). The main aim is to retain high levels of content validity but to increase standardization and objectivity.

Research outcomes

The historical overview shows the developments that have taken place in the assessment of clinical competence in the last few decades. The aspiration to develop test methods reflecting real-life professional tasks, together with the increasing awareness that assessment methods drive learning and education, have been central issues in this evolution. Most of these developments were associated with empirical research. The outcomes of this research will be discussed below, focusing on two aspects: first, the most prominent findings related to reliability and validity; second, findings associated with the effect of assessment on student learning.

Reliability and validity

It is not the intention here to go into detail about the research concerned
with each of the methods listed in Figure 8.1. Instead, the most consistent
and dominating outcomes from research conducted in the last decades
will be summarized. These consistencies may provide compelling direc-
tives for choices among methods for competence assessment.

Scores generalize poorly across test elements

This has been one of the most consistent findings in all competence
research. A score on one particular test item (i.e. a task, situation,
problem or case) is not very predictive for a score on another test item. In
other words, low correlations are found between test elements. Originally, this was documented in research on methods of problem-solving,
leading the investigators to conclude that problem-solving is a highly
content-specific ability (Elstein *et al.*, 1978). The low correlations between test elements present a significant problem to assessment. Generally, we wish to infer someone's competency from a test score,
irrespective of the particular sample of test elements given to the
examinee. If low correlations between test elements exist, then the
particular test elements used in one test will not be very predictive of
performance on a similar test constructed from a random selection of
items from the same pool of test elements. This problem has been called
the 'content specificity' problem.

Content specificity, however, is not unique for problem-solving instruments. It has been found for virtually all methods used for the assessment
of clinical competence including oral examinations (Swanson, 1987),
vignette-based short answer and menu tests (de Graaff *et al.*, 1987; Page
et al., 1990), chart-audits (Erviti *et al.*, 1980), performance-based tests
(van der Vleuten & Swanson, 1990*a*) and computer-based simulations
(Swanson *et al.*, 1987; Norcini & Swanson, 1989).

Content specificity turns out to be the most important source of error
influencing the reliability (generalizability) of examinations. Other
sources of variance (e.g. rater error; patient error) contribute much less
and can be dealt with more effectively (e.g. rater training; structured
marking sheets; standardized patients) (van der Vleuten *et al.*, 1991).

To achieve generalizable or stable scores (i.e. scores which are independent of the particular sample given) many test elements (cases,
problems, situations, stations) are required. The inevitable outcome of

Table 8.1. *Generalizability coefficients as a function of testing time for different methods varying in fidelity*

Where examiners/markers are involved, generalizability coefficients for a single examiner/marker per testing element are used

Testing time (hours)	MCQ[a]	Case-based short essays[b]	PMP[a]	Oral examination[c]	Multiple-station examination[d]
1	0.62	0.68	0.36	0.45	0.43
2	0.76	0.73	0.53	0.46	0.60
4	0.93	0.84	0.69	0.47	0.76
8	0.93	0.92	0.82	0.48	0.86

[a] Norcini *et al.*, 1985.
[b] Stalenhoef-Halling *et al.*, 1990.
[c] Swanson, 1987.
[d] Newble & Swanson, 1988.

this is prolonged testing time, so efficiency of test procedures becomes an important issue. The more efficient the format, the more generalizable the test scores and the less total testing time is needed.

Content specificity also poses a major problem because, unfortunately, fidelity and generalizability are inversely related to a large extent. Table 8.1 provides an illustration of the seriousness of the generalizability problem in relation to fidelity. It contains examples of reliability estimates reported in the literature for various instruments varying on the fidelity dimension. Reliability is expressed in terms of generalizability coefficients as a function of testing time. These coefficients can be interpreted similarly to the traditionally reported Cronbach's alpha (α). A value of 0.80 is considered generally a minimally acceptable value although higher values might be required for some purposes (e.g. certification). This is achieved in about two hours using MCQs, whether testing recall of isolated facts or testing application of this factual knowledge using patient vignettes. Almost twice as long is required to reach an acceptable value for multiple-station examinations. PMPs require about six to eight hours of testing time.

Scores do generalize across methods or testing formats

The literature on the assessment of clinical competence is rich with publications arguing that the method determines what is being measured. For example, MCQs are often criticized because of their limiting capacity to assess higher order cognitive skills. Other methods (e.g. open ended questions, oral examinations) are seen to be preferable because, by the nature of their qualities, they are able to assess more relevant dimensions of clinical competence. The empirical evidence, however, does not support this intuitive notion. On the contrary, many studies have documented high correlations (especially when corrected for unreliability due to content specificity, so-called true correlations) between scores on a wide variety of different methods, such as open-ended questions and MCQs (Norman *et al.*, 1987; Stalenhoef-Halling *et al.*, 1990; Schuwirth *et al.*, 1992), PMPs and MCQs (Norcini *et al.*, 1985), oral examinations, computer simulations and written tests (Maatsch, 1980, 1987; Maatsch & Huang, 1986), and between performance-based tests and multiple-choice tests (van der Vleuten *et al.*, 1989).

However, one should interpret these correlations with caution. High correlation between methods does not imply automatically that the methods measure the same thing. For example, length and weight of human beings are highly correlated, but they are clearly different entities. On the other hand, from a decision-making perspective, high correlation implies that relatively little unique information is gathered and that similar decisions can be made irrespective of the method used.

This research indicates, at the very least, that the boundaries between methods are not as solid as we tend to believe. The intuitive direct linkage between method used and competency being measured has been described as one of the most damaging myths in the assessment of clinical competence (McGuire, 1987). More important than the method itself is the content being measured within the method. The kind of task given to the examinee is the prime determinant of what is being measured. Naturally, not all tasks can be measured by all methods and there are well-known method–task interactions. It is, for instance, quite difficult or impossible to measure clinically important communication skills with written tests although other relevant clinical tasks could be designed into well-constructed written tests. Equally, open-ended questions focusing on facts only would measure no more than lower cognitive abilities.

Assessment drives learning

Many authors have indicated the close relationship that exists between the format and outcome of assessment and what students actually do (Entwistle, 1981; Newble & Jaeger, 1983; Frederiksen, 1984; Bouhuijs *et al.*, 1987; Stillman & Swanson, 1987; Newble, 1988; van der Vleuten *et al.*, 1989; Gibbs, 1992). For instance, Newble & Jaeger (1983) demonstrated that after the introduction of a performance-based clinical examination students spent more time learning clinical skills and less time preparing for theoretical examinations and this effect appeared to be enduring (Newble, 1988). Although the relationship between assessment and learning is well documented, little research has been conducted on its specific nature. More systematic study is required to determine precisely which effects are to be expected for which assessment strategies.

Implications for the choice of methods

The selection of methods is highly dependent on the context of the specific testing situation. For instance, quite different choices might be made for a high-stakes certification examination than for an in-training formative assessment. Moreover, method selection will be influenced by available resources (time, space, availability of clinical material, money), as well as tradition and personal or institutional preferences. A cookery-book solution to the selection of testing methods is therefore inappropriate. However, the research outcomes described in the previous section may provide some guidance.

Reliability issues

The reliability issues are concerned with the problem of content specificity and hence the efficiency of testing methods. In situations where high reliability is required and resources are limited, it may be necessary to select the most efficient testing method, perhaps at the expense of some other desirable test characteristic.

Without doubt, the most efficient test format is the MCQ. A suitable alternative may be short-answer questions, depending on the number of examinees and the availability of markers to score the answers. Other methods are more time consuming if reliability requirements are to be met (see Table 8.1). Therefore, efficiency clearly conflicts with fidelity and compromises have to be found. There are three possible strategies to be considered.

First, within a particular method, efficiency can be obtained by limiting time allocated for individual test elements (cases, stations, items). This will increase the number of elements that can be administered within the same examination period. One possible way of doing this without undue loss of fidelity is to restrict the assessment to the most critical issues as was discussed earlier in the 'key-features' approach. This approach has been applied successfully to written methods already but also could be used for other methods.

A second strategy is to use resources efficiently in order to increase testing time. If, for example, in a multiple-station examination the number of available examiners is limited, more can be gained, in terms of reliability, by having one examiner per station and increasing the number of stations than can be gained by improving rater reliability by having two examiners per station (van der Vleuten & Swanson, 1990*b*). Any additional error arising from examiner bias will be averaged out across test elements.

Another efficiency strategy is to use a sequential testing design. This makes use of the fact that tests which are not highly reliable can be used to identify the very high and very low scoring examinees. Thus, a relatively short screening test can be used for all examinees and those scoring high or low (distant from the pass/fail point) are excused from further testing. A subsequent, and more reliable, test is given to the remaining candidates to discriminate more accurately in the vicinity of the pass/fail point.

A third strategy is to combine efficient and less efficient methods into a test battery. From a validity perspective this is probably the preferred approach. However, care is needed when combining the scores from different test components (see Chapters 6 and 10).

Whatever strategy is followed it is clear that to achieve generalizable scores for assessments of clinical competence more testing time is needed than one assumes intuitively and one encounters in current practice. Even the most efficient testing methods will require at least three hours of testing time. With other methods the situation becomes considerably worse and test-length requirements of at least one day are not an exception (Swanson 1987; Swanson *et al.*, 1987; Norcini & Swanson, 1989; van der Vleuten & Swanson, 1990*a*). It should also be clear that an unreliable method can have no validity. Therefore, the choice of methods will be influenced strongly by its reliability characteristics.

Validity issues

An essential implication of what has been discussed is that we should discontinue attempts to classify and to rank-order methods in terms of their validity for measuring particular aspects or components of competence. The validity of a method does not exist. Validity can be established only through the relevance of the content represented in the kind of tasks given to the examinee, (see Chapters 6 and 7). As a consequence, irrespective of the method, the issue is how to construct and to select relevant tasks. The most relevant tasks are probably those reflecting reality as closely as possible. Nevertheless, not all methods are appropriate for assessing all tasks and informed selection is necessary.

The potential advantages of this approach are substantial. At present, it is difficult to obtain agreement on the definition of clinical competence and which attributes or components should be measured. It is much easier to have discussions focused on the relevance of clinical tasks and to relate this back to the educational programme or to the professional context. Instead of debating abstract concepts, one is discussing concrete examples of expected competence or performance.

In the past, the literature on the validity of educational tests has favoured indirect procedures, usually based on experimental correlation studies (Cronbach, 1960, 1983, 1988). Mainly, such procedures have developed from theoretical psychological research. Ebel (1961, 1983) has argued that educational tests are quite different from psychological tests, because in the former the content has direct significance. For validation of educational tests, direct methods seem to be more appropriate. These include the delineation of content categories, the use of blueprints, sampling problems over content categories and translating tasks into scores (see Chapter 6). Unfortunately, the value of using direct validation techniques to judge the quality of clinical competence assessments is not reflected in the literature, where indirect approaches continue to dominate.

The impact of the recent psychological research on medical expertise is more theoretical than practical at present. It does, however, stress the importance of knowledge structured in its clinical context and is in accord with the previous messages of having to be concerned about clinical content and fidelity. It also emphasizes the value of using direct validation techniques as proposed by Ebel (1961, 1983). Possibly, new test methods will arise from this understanding, which will discriminate more efficiently and validly between the competent and incompetent.

Impact on student learning issues

Reference has already been made to the enormous impact of assessment on student learning and behaviour. Yet, on the whole, medical teachers focus on the teaching aspects of the educational programme with little time being spent on assessment procedures. The side effects of this neglect are very obvious but recognized rarely. Newble & Jaeger (1983), in the study quoted previously, showed how well-considered alterations to assessment procedures, introduced as part of a major curriculum revision, produced changes in student behaviour which were the exact antithesis of that intended by the faculty. The study also showed that further alterations to student assessment rectified the situation without modification of the teaching programme. Another example of unexpected side-effects was reported by van Luijk *et al.*, (1990). A performance-based test was introduced and achieved the expected positive effects on clinical skills. Subsequently, students continued to score well, yet had obvious superficial understanding of the skills they were demonstrating. Then it was discovered that the students were memorizing the check-lists used by examiners in previous years. These tactics are similar to the well-recognized 'spotting' and 'cramming' that are associated with many written examinations.

Another aspect of the relationship between test format and student learning behaviour is illustrated by a study by van der Vleuten *et al.* (1989). They demonstrated that scores on a performance-based clinical test could be predicted very well by scores on a written test about clinical skills. In the past it might have been argued that the simple and cheap written test could replace the complex and costly performance-based test. (Indeed such arguments were used regularly in North America in the 1960s to replace traditional clinical examinations and essay tests with multiple-choice tests.) However, it is appreciated now that such a change would lead to the same effect as that found by Newble & Jaeger (1983) – students would prepare themselves differently by focusing on the theoretical aspects of the acquisition of clinical skills at the expense of the hands-on experience they would have undertaken to prepare for the performance-based test.

The message is clear: when choosing test methods, close attention must be given to their ability to deliver an assessment which is both valid and reliable. Equally close attention must be given to the potential and actual effects that test methods and assessment procedures have on student learning. They must be guiding students in the desired direction.

Acceptability issues

Although the issue of acceptability has not been discussed, it has been found to be critical. The literature contains many examples of research studies discrediting methods of assessment which, although they are in common usage, nevertheless continue to be used widely. A good example is the traditional clinical viva voce examination which was mainly discontinued in North America on the basis of research evidence of its unreliability. Yet is continues to be the backbone of clinical assessment in medical schools and colleges in the UK and Australasia. On the other hand, there are many examples of potentially valuable methods of assessment which have failed to advance beyond the experimental stage. If the quality of the assessment of clinical competence is to be improved recommendations must be made in a way which will be acceptable to the decision makers who determine policies and procedures.

Summary of suggestions for choice of methods

(i) Determine the tasks which are relevant to pose the examinees (and worry less about the competency being measured)

(ii) Select the tasks with the highest fidelity

(iii) Let the task dictate the method used and not vice versa

(iv) Select the method most capable of assessing the defined tasks and strive for efficiency within a given method

(v) Combine different methods into a battery of tests and use composite scores

(vi) Pay particular attention to the content of the examination and its translation to test scores and worry less about the theoretical validity of what is being measured

(vii) Verify the educational consequences of the method and aim to turn them to advantage

(viii) Verify the acceptability of the method

(ix) Evaluate the assessment procedure

Appendix: references relating to Figure 8.1

Assessment of clinical competence in general

Bender, W., Hiemstra, R., Scherpbier, A. & Zwierstra, R. (Eds.) (1990). *Teaching and Assessing Clinical Competence*. Groningen: BoekWerk Publications.
Hart I. & Harden, R. (Eds.) (1987). *Further Developments in Assessing Clinical Competence*. Montreal: Can-Heal Publications.
Hart, I., Harden, R. & Walton, H. (Eds.) (1987). *Newer Development in Assessing Clinical Competence*. Montreal: Can-Heal Publications.

Neufeld, V. & Norman, G. (Eds.) (1985). *Assessing Clinical Competence*. New
    York: Springer.
Norman, G., Allery, L., Berkson, L., Bordage, G., Cohen, R., Dauphinee,
    D., Davis, W., Friedman, C., Grant, J., Lear, P., Morris, P. & van der
    Vleuten, C. (1990). 'The psychology of clinical reasoning: implications for
    assessment'. *Paper presented at the Fourth Cambridge Conference.*
    Cambridge: Cambridge University School of Clinical Medicine.

Written Simulations

McGuire, C. (1987). Written methods for assessing clinical competence. In
    Further Developments in Assessing Clinical Competence, ed. I. R. Hart &
    R. M. Harden, pp. 44–58. Montreal: Can-Heal Publications.

PMP

McGuire, C. & Solomon, C. (1976). *Construction and Use of Written
    Simulations*. Chicago: The Psychological Corporation.

MEQ

Feletti, G. & Engel, C. (1980). The modified essay question for testing
    problem-solving skills. *Medical Journal of Australia*, **1**, 79–80.

P4-deck

Barrows, H. & Tamblyn, R. (1977). The portable patient problem pack (P4).
    A problem-based learning unit. *Journal of Medical Education*, **52**, 1002–4.

Computer simulations

CBX

Norcini, J., Meskauskas, J., Langdon, L. & Webster, G. (1986). An evaluation
    of a computer simulation in the assessment of physican competence.
    Evaluation in the Health Professions, **9**, 286–304.

CRT

Williams, R., Vu, N., Barrows, H. & Verhulst, S. (1984). Profile of the
    Clinical Reasoning Test (CRT): an objective measure of problem solving
    skills and proficiency in using medical knowledge. In *Tutorials in Problem-
    Based Learning*, ed. H. Schmidt & M. De Volder. Assen: Van Gorcum.

Key-features approach

Norman, G., Bordage, G., Currey, L., Dauphinee, D., Jolly, B., Newble, D.,
    Rothman, A., Stalenhoef, B., Stillman, P., Swanson, D. & Tonesk, X.
    (1985). A review of recent innovations in assessment. In *Directions in*

Clinical Assessment, ed. R. Wakeford, pp. 8–27. Cambridge: Cambridge University School of Clinical Medicine.

Q4

Bordage, G. & Page, G. (1987). An alternative approach to PMPs: the 'key features' concept. In *Further Developments in Assessing Clinical Competence*, ed. I. R. Hart & R. M. Harden, pp. 59–72. Montreal: Can-Heal Publications.

SIMP

de Graaff, E., Post, G. & Drop, M. (1987) Validation of a new measure of clinical problem-solving. *Medical Education*, **21**, 213–8.

Cognitive (psychological) measures

Norman, G. (1989) Reliability and construct validity of some cognitive measures of clinical reasoning. *Teaching and Learning in Medicine*, **1**, 194–9.

Pattern recognition

Case, S., Swanson, D. & Stillman, P. (1988) Evaluating diagnostic pattern recognition: the psychometric characteristics of a new item format. *Proceedings of the Twenty-seventh Annual Conference on Research in Medical Education (RIME)*. Washington: American Association of Medical Colleges.

Multiple probability estimate

van Rossum, H., Briek, E., Bender, W. & Meinders, A. (1990). The transfer effect of one single patent demonstration on diagnostic judgment of medical students: both better and worse. In *Teaching and Assessing Clinical Competence*, ed. W. Bender, R. Hiemstra, A. Scherpbier & R. Zwierstra, pp. 435–40. Groningen: BoekWerk Publications.

Learning process measures

Structured oral examination

Muzzin, L. & Hart, L. (1985). Oral examinations. In *Assessing clinical Competence*, ed. V. Neufeld & G. Norman. New York: Springer.

Triple jump exercise

Powles, A., Wintrup, N., Neufeld, V., Wakefield, J., Coates, G. & Burrows, J. (1981). The triple jump exercise: further studies of an evaluative technique. *Proceedings of the Twentieth Annual Conference on Research in Medical Education.* Washington: American Association of Medical Colleges.

Performance-based tests

OSCE

Harden, R. & Gleeson, F. (1979). Assessment of clinical competence using an objective structured clinical examination (OSCE). *Medical Education*, **13**, 41–54.
Newble, D. (1988) Eight years' experience with a structured clinical examination. *Medical Education, 22*, 200–4.

Standardized patient-based testing

Stillman, P., Ruggill, J., Rutala, P. & Sabers, D. (1980). Patient instructors as teachers and evaluators. *Journal of Medical Education*, **55**, 186–93.

Effect of examinations on student learning

Frederiksen, N. (1984). The real test bias: influences of testing on teaching and learning. *American Psychologist*, **39**, 193–202.
Newble, D. & Jaeger, K. (1983). The effect of assessments and examinations on the learning of medical students. *Medical Education*, **17**, 165–71.
(See also references for OSCE and TJE.)

Progress test

van der Vleuten, C. & Verwijnen, G. (1990). A system for student assessment. In *Perspectives from the Maastricht Experience*, ed C. van der Vleuten & W. Wijnen. Amsterdam: Thesis-publication.

References

Bordage, G. & Page, G. (1987). An alternative approach to PMPs: The 'key features' concept. In *Further Developments in Assessing Clinical Competence*, ed. I. R. Hart & R. M. Harden, pp. 59–72. Montreal: Can-Heal Publications.

Bouhuijs, P., van der Vleuten, C. & van Luijk, S. (1987) The OSCE as a part of a systematic skills training approach. *Medical Teacher*, 9, 183–91.

Case, S., Swanson, D. & van der Vleuten, C. (1991). Strategies for student assessment. In *The Challenge of Problem-based Learning*, ed. D. Boud, & G. Feletti, pp. 260–73. London: Kogan Page.

Cronbach, L. (1960). Validity. In *Encyclopedia of Educational Research*, ed. C. Harris, pp. 1551–5. New York: MacMillan.

Cronbach, L. (1983) What price simplicity? *Educational Measurement: Issues and Practice*, 2, 11–12.

Cronbach, L. (1988). Five perspectives on validity argument. In *Test Validity*, ed. H. Wainer & H. Braun, pp. 3–17. Hillsdale, NJ: Lawrence Erlbaum.

de Graaff, E., Post, G. & Drop, M. (1987). Validation of a new measure of clinical problem-solving. *Medical Education*, 21, 213–8.

Ebel, R. (1961). Must all tests be valid? *American Psychologist*, 16, 640–7.

Ebel, R. (1983) The practical validation of tests of ability. *Educational Measurement: Issues and Practice*, 2, 7–10.

Elstein, A., Shulman, L. & Sprafka, S. (1978). *Medical Problem Solving An Analysis of Clinical Reasoning*. Harvard University Press: Cambridge Massachusetts.

Entwistle, N. (1981). *Styles of Learning and Teaching*. Chichester: John Wiley & Sons.

Erviti, V., Templeton, B., Bunce, J. & Burg, F. (1980). The relationships of pediatric resident recording behavior across medical conditions. *Medical Care*, 18, 1020–31.

Fabb, W. & Marshall, J. (1983). *The Assessment of Clinical Competence in General Family Practice*. Lancaster: MTP Press.

Frederiksen, N. (1984). The real test bias: influences of testing on teaching and learning. *American Psychologist*, 39, 193–202.

Friedman, R., Korst, D., Schultz, J., Beatty, E. & Entine, S. (1978). Experience with the simulated patient physician encounter. *Journal of Medical Education*, 53, 825–30.

Gibbs, G. (1992). *Improving the Quality of Student Learning*. Bristol: Technical & Educational Services.

Grant, J. & Marsden, P. (1988). Primary knowledge, medical education, and consultant expertise. *Medical Education*, 22, 746–53.

Harden, R. & Gleeson, F. (1979) Assessment of clinical competence using an objective structured clinical examination (OSCE). *Medical Education*, 13, 41–54.

Maatsch, J. (1980). *Model for a Criterion-Referenced Medical Specialty Test*. Final Report Grant No. HS-02038-02, Office of Medical Education Research and Development, Michigan State University.

Maatsch, J. (1987). 'Theories of clinical competence: the construct validity of objective tests and performance assessments'. Paper presented at the International Conference on Evaluation in Medical Education, Beer Sheva, Israel, May 25–28.

Maatsch, J. & Huang, R. (1986). An evaluation of the construct validity of four alternative theories of clinical competence. *Proceedings of the Twenty-fifth Annual Conference on Research in Medical Education*. Washington: American Association of Medical Colleges.

McGuire, C. (1987). Written methods for assessing clinical competence. In *Further Developments in Assessing Clinical Competence*, ed. I. R. Hart & R. M. Harden, pp. 44–58. Montreal: Can-Heal Publications.

McLeskey, C. & Ward, R. (1978). Validity of written examinations. *Anesthesiology*, **49**, 224.

Neufeld, V. & Norman, G. (Eds.) (1985). *Assessing Clinical Competence*. New York: Springer.

Newble, D. (1988). Eight years' experience with a structured clinical examination. *Medical Education*, **22**, 200–4.

Newble, D. & Jaeger, K. (1983). The effect of assessments and examinations on the learning of medical students. *Medical Education*, **17**, 165–71.

Newble, D. & Swanson, D. (1988). Psychometric characteristics of the objective structured clinical examination. *Medical Education*, **22**, 325–34.

Norcini, J. & Swanson, D. (1989). Factors influencing testing time requirements for simulation-based measurements: do simulations ever yield reliable scores? *Teaching and Learning in Medicine*, **1**, 85–91.

Norcini, J., Swanson, D., Grosso, L., Shea, J. & Webster, G. (1985). Reliability, validity and efficiency of multiple choice question and patient management problem item formats in the assessment of physician competence. *Medical Education*, **19**, 238–47.

Norman, G. (1989). Reliability and construct validity of some cognitive measures of clinical reasoning. *Teaching and Learning in Medicine*, **1**, 194–9.

Norman, G., Allery, L., Berkson, L., Bordage, G., Cohen, R., Dauphinee, D., Davis, W., Friedman, C., Grant, J., Lear, P., Morris, P. & van der Vleuten, C. (1990). 'The psychology of clinical reasoning: implications for assessment' *Paper Presented at the Fourth Cambridge Conference*. Cambridge: Cambridge University School of Clinical Medicine.

Norman, G., Bordage, G., Curry, L., Dauphinee, D., Jolly, B., Newble, D., Rothman, A., Stalenhoef, B., Stillman, P., Swanson, D. & Tonesk, X. (1985). A review of recent innovations in assessment. In *Directions in Clinical Assessment*, ed. R. Wakeford, pp. 8–27. Cambridge: Cambridge University School of Clinical Medicine.

Norman, G., Smith, E., Powles, A., Rooney, P., Henry, N. & Dodd, P. (1987). Factors underlying performance on written tests of knowledge. *Medical Education*, **2**, 297–304.

Page, G., Bordage, G., Harasym, P., Bowmer, I. & Swanson, D. (1990). A revision of the Medical Council of Canada's qualifying examination: pilot test results. In *Teaching and Assessing Clinical Competence*, ed. W. Bender, R. Hiemstra, A. Scherpbier & R. Zwierstra, pp. 403–7. Groningen: BoekWerk Publications.

Schmidt, H., Norman, G. & Boshuizen, H. (1990). A cognitive perspective on medical expertise: theory and implications. *Academic Medicine*, **65**, 611–21.

Schuwirth, L., van der Vleuten, C. & Donkers, H. (1992). Het gebruik van open en gesloten vragen: effecten van cueing en nauwkeurigheid van computergestuurde scoring. (The use of open-ended and objective questions: cueing effects and precision of computer-based scoring.) In *Gezond Onderwijs* I, ed. C. van der Vleuten, A. Scherpbier & M. Pollemans, pp. 312–18. Houten: Bohn, Stafleu, Van Loghum.

Stalenhoef-Halling, B., van der Vleuten, C., Jaspers, T. & Fiolet, J. (1990). The feasibility, acceptability and reliability of open-ended questions in a problem-based learning curriculum. In *Teaching and Assessing Clinical Competence*, ed. W. Bender, R. Hiemstra, A. Scherpbier & R. Zwierstra, pp. 552–7. Groningen: BoekWerk Publications.

Stillman, P. & Swanson, D. (1987). Ensuring the clinical competence of medical school graduates through standardized patients. *Archives of Internal Medicine*, **147**, 1049–52.

Swanson, D. (1987). A measurement framework for performance-based tests. In *Further Developments in Assessing Clinical Competence*, ed. I. Hart & R. M. Harden, pp. 13–36. Montreal: Can-Heal Publications.

Swanson, D., Norcini, J. & Grosso, L. (1987). Assessment of clinical competence: written and computer-based simulations. *Assessment and Evaluation in Higher Education*, **12**, 220–46.

van der Vleuten, C. & Swanson, D. (1990*a*). Assessment of clinical skills with standardized patients: state of the art. *Teaching and Learning in Medicine*, **2**, 58–76.

van der Vleuten, C. & Swanson, D. (1990*b*). Five strategies for reducing resource requirements for tests involving standardized patients. In *Teaching and Assessing Clinical Competence*, ed. W. Bender, R. Hiemstra, A. Scherpbier & R. Zwierstra, pp. 344–51. Groningen: BoekWerk Publications.

van der Vleuten, C. & Verwijnen, G. (1990). Assessment in problem-based learning. In *Problem-based Learning Perspectives from the Maastricht Approach*, ed. C. van der Vleuten & W. Wijnen. Amsterdam: Thesis Publication.

van der Vleuten, C., Norman, G. & de Graaff, E. (1991). Pitfalls in the pursuit of objectivity: issues of reliability. *Medical Education*, **25**, 110–8.

van der Vleuten, C., van Luijk, S. & Beckers, H. (1989). A written test as an alternative to performance testing. *Medical Education*, **23**, 97–107.

van Luijk, S., van der Vleuten, C. & van Schelven, R. (1990). The relation between content and psychometric characteristics in performance-based testing. In *Teaching and Assessing Clinical Competence*, ed. W. Bender, R. Hiemstra, A. Scherpbier & R. Zwierstra, pp. 202–7. Groningen: BoekWerk Publications.

Wakeford, R. (Ed.) (1985). *Directions in Clinical Assessment*. Cambridge: Cambridge University School of Clinical Medicine.

9

Standard setting in certification tests

IAN BOWMER (Editor), WAYNE DAVIS,
JACQUES DES MARCHAIS, ROGER GABB,
JOHN NORCINI and GREGORY WHELAN

The conceptualization of competence is not only the right of every profession, it is also its responsibility. A profession is defined when society recognizes a circumscribed and distinct body of knowledge. The profession sets the standards of competency and the level of performance expected. Certification represents the recognition that the standard of competency has been achieved.

Historically, certifying bodies have been accountable only to themselves for their actions. In medicine, the high esteem in which doctors were held gave an unparalleled level of autonomy from the community in determining who was suitable to practise. With society's increasing requirement for accountability, certifying bodies are being asked to justify their actions. Although courts of law will not normally challenge the knowledge content of a profession, the procedures by which professions allow entry into their ranks are scrutinized increasingly.

Standard setting and the assessment process must not only be reasonable and consistent, but also must appear to be so. There is a need to avoid criticism concerned with issues of equity where discrimination is based potentially on school of graduation, ethnic origin or sex, rather than knowledge and skill. In Australia, this has led to the establishment of the National Office of Overseas Skills Recognition which is developing explicit competency-based standards for the professions (Gonczi *et al.*, 1990). Relman (1988) notes that critics also demand explicit standards to prevent a professional group from setting unnecessarily high standards in order to control competition or to reduce the standards to force practitioners into underserviced areas.

Standard setting can be defined as the process used by a professional body to define a level of performance based on various assessment measures or test instruments. An individual must demonstrate performance at this level to be judged competent. Certification recognizes this performance.

The standard-setting process

The standard to be used cannot be determined until there is agreement on the purpose of the test. To reach this agreement, the level of the candidates must be identified clearly and the domains to be tested need to be defined.

Who sets the standard? For both statistical and political reasons, the standard setting must be fair and seen to be unbiased. This requires multiple judgements from a broad sample of the professional community who have intimate knowledge of the performance required of the candidates. To avoid bias, those responsible for the test development should be excluded. For the medical profession, the composition should include both academic and non-academic practitioners, urban and rural practitioners, members of minorities and majorities, and of both sexes. Members of the general public, while ensuring the process is fair and follows a set procedure, would not participate in the actual judgements.

Methodology

A standard is the score that separates those who pass from those who fail. It is an answer to the question, 'How much is enough?' (Livingston & Zieky, 1982). There are two kinds of standards: relative and absolute. Relative standards are based on a comparison among examinees. For instance, a standard that passes the top 90% of examinees is a relative standard. Absolute standards are independent of the performance of examinees; they are expressed in terms of how much an examinee needs to know. For example, an absolute standard is one that would pass all examinees who respond correctly to more than 70% of the test questions.

Regardless of whether they are relative or absolute, all standards are arbitrary (Glass, 1978). Because competence as a doctor is distributed continuously, examinees do not sort themselves neatly into competent and incompetent groups. Consequently, exactly where the standard is placed in the distribution of scores is subjective. Moreover, selection of a standard is always based on human judgement and it is, therefore, subject to all the factors that influence such judgements. Some of the specific factors that influence standards are the method used to set them, the particular judges who are involved in the process and social needs when the standard is set. Although standards are arbitrary, they need not be capricious (Popham, 1978). They can be set using processes that render defensible judgements, and such judgements are needed by society (e.g. society needs to know who is qualified as a surgeon or as a specialist physician (internist)).

Who should set standards

A key part of making defensible judgements is selection of the appropriate number and type of judges. In general, it is best to set standards in a group of at least 10 members. There are instances, however, when fewer members, working away from the meeting, or several different groups working on different parts of the test are responsible alternatives (Norcini *et al.*, 1987; Norcini *et al.*, 1988*b*). The judges should be knowledgeable in the field of the examination and, for the sake of credibility, some should be experts or leaders in the field. If it is an examination for entry into a profession, it would also be helpful to include educators who are familiar with the training process and the level of ability of those completing training. This ensures that the most knowledgeable group sets the standard, and it provides credibility with the examinees and the public.

Relative standard-setting methods

Fixed percentage method

The most straightforward of the relative standard-setting methods is the fixed percentage method. A group of judges is identified and they begin their meeting by discussing the purpose of the examination and the characteristics of the examinees. This should be followed by a thorough review of the content of the test and, where appropriate, it is advisable for the group to take the test as the examinees would.

At the end of this exercise, the group members announce aloud what percentage of examinees they expect to pass. These percentages are copied onto a flip chart or blackboard and the judges with the highest and lowest percentages lead a discussion. Throughout this discussion, the judges should have the opportunity to change their estimates. When the exchange is completed, the percentages are averaged to derive the pass rate.

Reference group method

In the reference group method, a subgroup of examinees is identified and a fixed percentage is passed. The score that separates those who pass from those who fail in this subgroup is then applied to all other examinees. For instance, the American Board of Internal Medicine (ABIM) had a reference group composed of all USA medical school graduates who were taking the examination for the first time and had finished residency training in the year of the examination. The ABIM decided that the top 84% of this group should pass (the mean minus one standard deviation). Therefore, the score that separated the top 84% of the reference group from the bottom 16% was the cutting score, and all other examinees (e.g. repeat takers of the examination) needed to achieve this score in order to pass. Application of this method is identical to the fixed percentage method, except that a reference needs to be identified as part of the initial group discussion.

Pros and cons of relative standard-setting methods

Relative standard-setting methods are sensitive to examinee perform-ance, but are not necessarily sensitive to the relevance of the test itself (i.e. although not recommended, the standard could be set without even looking at the examination). Such methods are easy to implement, compute and explain to the examinees. However, they may not be quite as credible as absolute standards.

The fixed percentage method is most useful when the top examinees are to be selected. For instance, if there is a limit on the number of admissions to a medical school, this method may be among the better alternatives. The reference group method is most useful when a particu-lar group of examinees is very well known to the standard setters and some fixed percentage is expected to be qualified.

Relative standards have four shortcomings. First, the standards can fluctuate over time depending on the ability of the examinees. For example, the ABIM used the reference group method for a number of years while the ability of the group was slipping (Norcini *et al.*, 1989). As a consequence, the ABIM's standard slipped as well (i.e. it became easier to pass the examination). Second, relative standards may be viewed by some as an attempt to manipulate manpower, rather than to make a judgement about competence. Third, it is less appealing for examinees to be judged against the performance of others than it is to be judged against an absolute standard based on the quality of a performance. Fourth, some examinees will fail regardless of how much test material they know.

Absolute standard-setting methods

Several methods are available to set absolute standards (see also Chapter 6). Many are variations on the methods described by Angoff (1971) and Ebel (1972). As a consequence, these two will be described. Details concerning variations on the techniques or other methods can be found elsewhere (Livingston & Zieky, 1982; Berk, 1986).

Angoff's method

As with the relative standard-setting methods, a group of judges is convened and they begin their meeting by discussing the purpose of the examination and the characteristics of the examinees. Again, this should be followed by a thorough review of the content of the test and, when appropriate, the group should take the test as the examinees would.

Angoff's method involves making judgements about how a borderline group of examinees will answer each item. At the start of the exercise, the judges need to discuss the characteristics of this borderline examinee. In doing so, they may find it helpful to think of all the examinees with whom they have been acquainted. Of this group, some (probably the majority) were clearly qualified to pass the examination and some (probably a small number) were clearly not qualified to pass. Those remaining, the ones about whom the judges were uncertain, constitute the borderline group. As the judges discuss the characteristics of this group, it is important for them to keep the purpose of the test in mind. For instance, a medical certifying examination is primarily a test of medical knowledge and judgement. Consequently, issues such as ethics and patient rapport should not be part of the considerations of a borderline group.

The major task of the meeting is to gather estimates of the proportion of the borderline group that will respond correctly to each question. The easier the question, the higher the estimate will be. The proportion must be between 0 and 1.0 and ordinarily should be at least as large as the chance of guessing the correct answer. For example, for a single-best-answer item with five options, the lowest proportion should be 0.20. After initial estimates are made by each member of the group, a discussion led by those giving the highest and lowest estimates should take place. All members of the group are then given an opportunity to review their initial estimate. This process is repeated for each item. Proportions assigned by each member of the group are averaged for each item and then summed over all items to arrive at a cutting score.

Ebel's method

This method also involves a group of judges estimating the performance of a borderline group of examinees. Consequently, the meeting begins the same way as the meeting for Angoff's method. However, the major task of the meeting is different. First, the judges must sort items into a two-dimensional array where one dimension is item relevance (essential, important, acceptable, questionable) and the other dimension is item difficulty (easy, medium, hard). For example, one item might be classified as easy and essential, while another might be classified as hard and acceptable.

Once all items have been classified into these 12 categories (4 relevance categories × 3 difficulty categories = 12 categories), the judges estimate the proportion of items that the borderline examinees will answer correctly for the first category. After initial estimates are made by each member of the group, a discussion is led by those giving the highest and lowest estimates, with judges being free to change their estimates at any time. This process is repeated for each of the 12 categories. Proportions assigned by each member of the group are averaged for each category, multiplied by the number of items in the category, and then summed over all categories to arrive at a cutting score.

Pros and cons of absolute standard-setting methods

Absolute standard-setting methods are sensitive to the relevance of the test, but they are not necessarily sensitive to the performance of examinees. As with relative methods, they are easy to implement, compute and explain to the test-takers, and are more defensible and credible than relative standards.

Use of absolute standard-setting methods is appropriate when mastery of content is involved and the percentage of qualified examinees is unknown. As a consequence, these methods are suited particularly to licensure and certification exams. They are less useful when a limited number of candidates who pass is desired.

These methods do have some limitations. The concept of the borderline group is foreign to some judges; they have difficulty identifying it and determining exactly how they think these examinees will perform on individual items. This is particularly true for experts, since they may have unrealistically high expectations and little experience with less qualified examinees. Less seriously, the task of assigning each item a value, or a category, is time consuming and it can be tedious.

Some tips for using absolute standards

  (i) If the judges are unfamiliar with the examination, they should take it before the meeting, which helps to prevent unrealistically high standards
 (ii) During the meeting, the judges should have access to the correct answers, which helps to prevent embarrassment and unrealistically low standards
(iii) Where possible, the judges should be given examinee performance data, which provides a 'reality check' and is especially necessary if the distribution of items is skewed (Norcini *et al.*, 1988*a*).
 (iv) Throughout the meeting, judges should be provided with data on the consequence of their decisions (i.e. projected pass rates)
  (v) All judges should attend the meeting, which gives them the feedback they require about how their standards and expectations compare with others
 (vi) If many items need to be assigned to categories or to be judged, the experts can do 30–40 items in the group (or as many as needed to calibrate their judgements) and the remainder can be completed at home (Norcini *et al.*, 1987, 1988*b*)

Summary

Standard setting is the responsibility of every professional organization and requires clear definition of the body of knowledge and clear expectations of the practitioner. The use of a normative process to set the standard can no longer be considered to be acceptable within professional bodies. The use of defined performance criteria within the professional context is the only fair and equitable mechanism of judging competence. Judgements should be made by a broad group of the profession who are instructed about the process and provided with feedback of candidate's performance. The definition of the level of performance must be understood by all judges, since the range of performance can be extensive. With careful training and follow-up, judgements can be demonstrated to be reliable and appropriate. Standard setting using this process can be defended by the profession in the legal arena (Cavanaugh, 1991) and has the potential to provide internationally acceptable criteria.

References

Angoff, W. H. (1971). Scales, norms and equivalent scores. In *Educational Measurement*, ed. R. L. Thorndike, pp. 508–600. Washington, DC: American Council on Education.

Berk, R. A. (1986). A consumer's guide to setting performance standards on criterion-referenced tests. *Review of Educational Research*, **56**, 137–72.

Cavanaugh, S. H. (1991). Response to a legal challenge. *Evaluation and the Health Professions*, **14**, 13–4.

Ebel, R. L. (1972). *Essentials of Educational Measurement*. Englewood Cliffs, NJ: Prentice-Hall.

Glass, G. V. (1978). Standards and criteria. *Journal of Educational Measurement*, **15**, 237–61.

Gonczi, A., Hager, P. & Oliver, L. (1990). *Establishing Competency Based Standards in the Professions*. National Office of Overseas Skills Recognition Research Paper No. 1. Canberra: Australian Government Publishing Service.

Livingston, S. A. & Zieky, M. J. (1982). *Passing Scores: A Manual for Setting Standards of Performance on Educational and Occupational Tests*. Princeton: Educational Testing Service.

Norcini, J. J., Lipner, R. S., Langdon, L. O. & Strecker, C. A. (1987). A comparison of three variations on a standard-setting method. *Journal of Educational Measurement*, **24**, 56–64.

Norcini, J. J., Maihoff, N. A., Day, S. C. & Benson, J. A., Jr (1989). Trends in medical knowledge as assessed by the certifying examination in Internal Medicine. *Journal of the American Medical Association*, **262**, 2402–4.

Norcini, J. J., Shea, J. A. & Kanya, T. D. (1988*a*). The effect of various factors on standard-setting. *Journal of Educational Measurement*, **25**, 57–65.

Norcini, J. J., Shea, J. A. & Ping, J. C. (1988*b*). A note on the application of multiple matrix sampling to standard-setting. *Journal of Educational Measurement*, **25**, 159–64.

Popham, W. J. (1978). As always, provocative. *Journal of Educational Measurement*, **15**, 297–300.

Relman, A. S. (Editorial) (1988). Assessment and accountability: the third revolution in medical care. *New England Journal of Medicine*, **319**, 1220–2.

10

Combining components of assessment

JOHN FOULKES (Editor), RAJA
BANDARANAYAKE, RICHARD HAYS, GARRY
PHILLIPS, ARTHUR ROTHMAN, LESLEY
SOUTHGATE and RICHARD WAKEFORD

It is common practice to administer examinations which are combinations of assessment tasks. An obvious example is the summing of scores on a written test and on a clinical test to form an overall score. This chapter considers the rationale, implications and permissible ways of combining such scores.

Components of assessment

Examinations are designed usually so that their components are clearly visible. The components will have unique titles (such as 'Paper 1', 'Oral' and so on) and will occupy separate spaces on the examination timetable. The boundaries of each component are determined usually by the objectives of that component.

In some instances the boundaries may not be clear. There may be good administrative reasons for having a three-hour multiple-choice test which is composed of different sections in order to allow all responses to be made on a single answer sheet which could be read by a scanner. The sections of the test might, however, be different in respect of the subject matter tested; and different parts of the examination might contain tasks which test the same subject matter but in a different mode, such as an essay paper. 'Components', in a system such as this, might therefore be composed after the fact by the addition of part scores from various tests, in a way that may not be apparent to the candidates. An example of such an examination is that of the Royal Australian College of General

Practitioners. Components are defined therefore as whatever generates a unique (discrete) score, whether by content, skill area (domain) or test method.

The reasons for the use of more than one component differ somewhat according to the purpose of the examination, discussed below, but are explained essentially by the fact that most of the attributes examined are complex. The history of psychological testing shows that, for example, early attempts to devise intelligence tests soon stumbled over the problem of what is meant by intelligence and, subsequently, separate measures of verbal comprehension, associative memory, spatial reasoning, etc. were developed. In educational testing in medicine, it is commonly thought necessary to have different tests for theoretical and practical abilities.

In general, the ability which is to be examined is thought to consist of facets which are sufficiently different so that the possession of one does not guarantee possession of the others, with the result that all must be included in the assessment. At least, they must be assessed if it is practical to do so. However, the aims of a course of study typically include elements which are not examined, such as the development of attitudes.

The purpose of examinations

It is usual to classify examinations into categories such as achievement and aptitude, and so on, according to the purpose they are designed to serve. In fact, the sort of classification referred to here is not a very rigid one. The distinction between achievement and aptitude is often unclear. Examinations which are designed to be measures of achievement for school children may be used by institutions of higher education as the dominant factor in deciding whether to admit an applicant; they are apparently treating the examinations as if they were measures of aptitude. Nor is this necessarily wrong: a measure of achievement may indeed prove also to be a good measure of aptitude.

At the theoretical level at least, the distinction is important and the following discussion considers separately tests whose main purpose is the assessment of either aptitude or achievement. We recognize that the primary purposes of examining in medical education are certification or licensing. Consequently, the majority of examining in the field is to assess achievement, and some explanation must be offered of the space given over to aptitude testing in this chapter. The intention is to juxtapose the two approaches in order to clarify some of the less straightforward issues which arise in achievement testing. It should not be supposed that one approach is better than the other nor is it applicable to every situation.

Aptitude tests: the choice of components

Aptitude tests are judged by the accuracy with which they predict some outcome measure, which is termed the 'criterion'. The criterion itself may be a form of test, such as an assessment made after a further period of education or training, for which the candidate has shown aptitude in the original test. The criterion may also be some less precise measure, such as 'How good a family doctor is this person?', in which case the 'measure' is likely to be a combination of pieces of evidence, including judgemental evidence.

In most practical situations, the criterion will be complex. The good family doctor needs a range of disparate abilities. The aptitude test needs to take account of the complexity of the criterion and reflect it in the choice of components.

The task of predicting one performance from another can be expressed mathematically as a regression equation. In its simplest form, it is the equation for a straight line:

$$Y = a + bX$$

where X, in this context, is the aptitude test score, which is known, and Y is the criterion measure, which is to be predicted. The term b in the equation indicates how much Y increases for every increase in X; this is termed the regression weight and will be discussed in more detail below. The term a is a constant value which is added to the aptitude test score X in order to ensure that the mean predicted criterion score will be equal to the mean aptitude test score (Guilford & Fruchter, 1986).

In the discussion above, the aptitude test is conceived as consisting of a single component, designated X. If, as is more usual, the aptitude measure consists of more than one component, designated X_1, X_2, X_3 and so on, the problem in mathematical terms becomes one of multiple regression, and the equation may be written as follows:

$$Y = a + bX_1 + cX_2 + dX_3 + \ldots$$

for as many components as there are, each of which has its own weight: b, c, d and so on.

In order to determine the regression weights and the constant a, it is necessary to develop and administer some aptitude tests and wait until the criterion measures become available. Then, with X and Y known, the unknown values a, b, c and d can be calculated and used to predict the criterion score for future candidates for the aptitude test. The accuracy of the prediction will be seen to depend to some extent on the nature of the group of candidates who provide the data for the calculation of the regression weights.

The mathematical notation may be misleading in implying that the unknown quantity Y can be derived from the aptitude score X. In fact, the equation yields a predicted value of the criterion which is subject to error. This is hardly surprising: nothing is likely to be very accurate when measures of human behaviour are involved. It is possible to quantify the error; to say, in effect, that one score can be predicted from another, subject to a certain tolerance or margin of error. This margin of error depends on the closeness of the relationship between aptitude score and criterion score. If the correlation between the two is strong, the errors involved in predicting one from the other will be small; a weak correlation will lead to large errors in prediction.

Prediction can be improved by adding components to the aptitude test. The multiple regression equation that is set out above may lead to smaller errors in predicting Y than is the case with the simpler form of the equation in which there is only one component. This is understood intuitively from the fact that if the criterion is complex, more than one aptitude will have to be tested to serve as a basis for prediction. This provides a rationale for the use of multiple components in an aptitude test: the goal is to minimize the errors in prediction and therefore to save resources. There is a relatively simple mathematical procedure available to determine the value of potential components. A test development programme could be conducted by administering a vast array of disparate tests and then, when criterion scores become available, using multiple regression techniques to determine which tests provide the best prediction.

Decisions are not taken solely on the basis of the mathematics: a point will be reached where the addition of further tests improves the prediction only slightly, and probably at a cost which is not justified in terms of the improvement it brings to prediction and thus to cost savings elsewhere.

Decisions about which components to include in a battery of tests should also relate to issues such as the public perception of the test. It is to be expected that the content of the aptitude test will bear a reasonably obvious relationship or relevance to the criterion. If it transpires that some factor such as age, height or region of birth is a good predictor, it may not be acceptable on other grounds to include it as an aptitude measure.

Achievement tests: the choice of components

Achievement tests may appear to lack the theoretical framework that underlies aptitude tests and which has been set out briefly above. What theory could be said to govern the choice of what to examine in an achievement test?

If there is no theory, there are at least principles. As aptitude tests look to a future measure for their rationale, so achievement tests naturally look back to the courses of study of which they are the end point. The choice of the components to be included, and their relative importance, will be expected to show the influence of expert judgement, consensus, or contemporary wisdom, probably tempered by administrative consider-ations or constraints. To this extent the nature of the composite measure is defined by making judgements concerning the importance of the material assessed by each component. In such a case, subjective judge-ment is more valid than the use of empirical methods in the selection of components.

In operational terms, this has the consequence that achievement tests bearing identical titles may not be identical, since the designers of each will have arrived at a different 'definition' of the subject by the com-ponents they have chosen to include and by the relative importance attached to each. Further, a given achievement test changes over time, reflecting changing perceptions of the subject.

Achievement tests have both the ability to define a subject and the power to influence the course of study. An examination may lead the curriculum by the choice and weighting of components, which sends a clear message to those who are teaching the subject and those who are preparing themselves for the examination. On the other hand, teachers may influence examination authorities to ensure that the examinations reflect the curriculum and the way they teach.

Such principles have guided the development of achievement tests. However, other considerations, notably the mode of assessment or choice of assessment instrument, have had an influence. Many examin-ations now have a rather mixed structure. The written papers will often contain some form of objective test (most commonly, a multiple-choice paper) and some form of more traditional written test (e.g. a modification of the essay test). There may be some form of 'performance' test – practical, clinical or oral. There may also be an element of continuous assessment carried out locally but supervised from the centre. The influence of technology may be felt in some use of computers in the assessment. The general impression is of a process of accretion: the developers and administrators have added in test components which seemed like 'a good idea at the time'. Some erosion takes place, but the older forms of assessment, such as essays, have proved resilient and the newer forms have been added to them rather than replacing them entirely, so that examinations now are longer (or at least more complex in structure) than they were 30 years ago. This reluctance to replace has also resulted in duplication of methods used to test the same attribute.

Combining components: levels of measurement

Measurement is defined as 'the assignment of numerals or numbers to objects or events' and is made on one of four scales: nominal, ordinal, interval and ratio (Guilford & Fruchter, 1986, p. 21). These are arranged in a hierarchy, with nominal at the base and ratio at the top. Nominal refers to essentially category-based 'measurement', such as would be yielded by classifying people by sex, country of origin or type of employment and assigning a number to each category. Ordinal measurement is exemplified most obviously in assessment by rank ordering: first, second, third. Ordinal measurement uses numbers, but only for the purpose of ranking; it could not be said (without further evidence) that the difference between the candidates ranked first and second was the same as that between those ranked second and third. This is the property of interval measurement, which uses cardinal rather than ordinal numbers, such that the difference between scores of 22 and 24 is the same as that between scores of 28 and 30; the intervals are the same. Ratio scales are distinguished from interval scales because they have an origin, usually zero, which represents nothing of the property or attribute measured. As a result comparisons can be made between points on the scale. Thus, for example, temperature is measured in degrees centigrade on an interval scale and not on a ratio scale, because it is not true to say that something which has a temperature of 100 degrees is twice as hot as something with a temperature of 50 degrees.

Measurements – in this case, scores on different components – may be combined only if they are from identical levels of measurement, and if they are expressed in identical units of measurement. (Percentages are an example of units of measurement. If component scores are to be combined, this should be done after all (or none) have been converted to percentages or to some other common unit.) Where different levels of measurement exist, they may be combined only if a downward adjustment takes place to achieve the same level for all measurements to be combined: that is, if ratio scales are treated as interval scales or if interval scales are treated as rank orders. Level of measurement must also be considered before any arithmetical operations are carried out on the scores: clearly, nominal and ordinal scales cannot be used to calculate a mean and standard deviation for example.

The many instruments of assessment have differing marking systems, including a simple pass/fail statement, percentage correct, ranking, assigning categories and rating scales. Each of these marking systems possesses different mathematical properties which must be recognized and understood before components are combined.

Measurement properties of available test formats

The majority of test formats currently in widespread use yield what are considered to be interval scores. Multiple-choice and other forms of objective tests are scored by summing the points awarded for each answer to produce total scores, a scale on which it is assumed that intervals are equal. Free-format written-response types (essays, modified essay questions, short answer) are usually marked according to answer keys and assigned a numerical mark. However, essay marking may be more subjective and the means by which an impression or judgement is converted to a number may not be explicit.

Similarly, scores on oral examinations are often essentially subjective assessments recorded as numbers. Examiners may work with an ordinal scale such as 'not satisfactory', 'satisfactory', 'good' and 'very good', providing judgements which are then converted to scores such as 30, 40, 50 and 60 before being combined with other components. Thus, an ordinal scale is upgraded to an interval scale in a way that may lack foundation. Structured marking systems for orals may improve objectivity and produce a score based on individual sections of the oral examination, which is closer to the interval level.

Rating scales call for special discussion, since the term is used to describe a variety of instruments with different measurement properties.

A rating scale with a small number of points, each anchored in behaviours, is a nominal scale if the anchor points are not arranged in some order representing a gradation of the attribute being measured. Scores from these cannot be combined with interval scores and may be manipulated only by cross-tabulation and frequency counts. Rating scales with a small number of points between two ends, indicating some ordering of marks, are ordinal scales, while those with a larger number of points (say, more than 12) are likely to be treated as interval scales, even though it is actually almost impossible to achieve equidistance in rating. Test developers must decide therefore what kind of rating scale is to be used, and use interval scales where the intent is combination with other component scores. When total scores are calculated on the basis of the mean of a number of ratings, the scores have interval properties. For example, in the case of an objective structured clinical examination (OSCE) the total score may be regarded as interval, even if individual stations have checklists requiring yes/no answers, therefore providing nominal or ordinal data.

The commonest level at which combination occurs is the interval level, because this permits more complex statistical manipulation. There is therefore a temptation to regard the product of any marking system as an interval scale and a likelihood that ordinal scales will be treated as interval scales. The extent of the error committed in these cases needs to be judged from the particular circumstances, and in many instances it is probably a theoretical rather than a practical concern. Discovery of the error may lead to a test development effort to create a more truly interval scale for the scoring of instruments such as essays and orals.

An issue in all test formats where there is more than one marker per test, such as essays, is how the individual scores of each marker are to be combined. A decision to average the scores implies that the scale is regarded as interval. The alternative of debating until consensus is reached makes no such assumption. If, however, markers use a common marking scheme, scores approach an interval scale.

Pass/fail rules in combined tests

The decision whether or not to combine components will determine the way in which results are reported. If scores are not combined at all, a candidate 'profile' results. There is, or was recently, a great attraction in the notion of a profile; anything that contained the word seemed to be a good thing. The argument in favour of profiling is the extra information which it seems to offer. Why merge all the component scores into one total when it would be of interest to know how the candidate performed in each component?

This, to revert to the notion of the purpose of an examination, may be requiring an examination to do something for which it was not designed. It is, in effect, to treat an achievement test as though it were a diagnostic test, designed to reveal relative strengths and weaknesses. Achievement tests can work as measures of aptitude and there is no reason why they should not have a diagnostic function; but, since generally they are not designed to do so, the onus should be on the user to justify interpreting achievement tests in this way.

Achievement tests which consist of several components are sometimes thought to examine the underlying knowledge or skills by a stratified random sampling method; each component forms a stratum and, within that, questions sample at random all the material which may be tested legitimately in that area. If this idea is taken seriously – and it has its opponents – then it is not permissible to decompose the composite. That composite reflects a 'snapshot' of performance in the whole range of skills or tasks; a truncated, possibly distorted view of performance would be gained by assessing components of competence in the disconnected way that is implied by profile reporting. Further, it would have to be shown that the psychometric characteristics of the individual components were good enough for them to be reported on separately.

On the other hand, if it is acceptable to treat components separately for reporting purposes, it is then possible to construct an examination on a 'unit-credit' basis. Credit is given for each component passed, and only failed components are resat at future sessions of the examination. (Profile reporting would seem to carry with it the notion of a pass/fail or grading decision on each component.)

Taken to this extreme, it is doubtful whether we should continue to use the term 'component', since each element now assumes the status of an examination in its own right, and what are being combined are probably not scores but pass/fail decisions. A less extreme position is to treat a combination of components as an entity, but nevertheless to require a minimum level of performance in each component. This practice has been termed by Torgerson (1958) the 'conjunctive' model, and is contrasted with the 'compensatory' model, in which performance in individual components is allowed to range over all possible scores (including the very low) provided that the aggregate score is high enough for a given grade to be awarded. A minimum level of performance or competence, often referred to as a 'hurdle', may be set on any or all the components to ensure competence in a particular skill or task. For example, should an anaesthetist be unable to demonstrate cardiopulmonary resuscitation, it may be argued that performance in other tasks is irrelevant and that performance on the examination as a whole, however excellent, should not merit a pass because of this one critical failing. The requirement that candidates should demonstrate minimum competence in components of a battery of tests may be applied both to aptitude and to achievement tests.

Newbould (1982) points out that 'the relative values of the cut-off scores of the components, which set the hurdles, have differential "bite" (hence weight) according to the "heights" set. A set of "high" hurdles will have a different weight in determining results from a set of "low" ones'.

Issues of validity and reliability

In the earlier discussion of the choice of components it was suggested that these might well need to be diverse in order to reflect the many facets of the criterion (in the terminology of aptitude tests) or of the subject/curriculum (for achievement tests). Concern may be felt at combining components of assessment, since it may appear that apples and oranges are being added together. Specifically, if poorly-correlated components are added together, what are the implications for the reliability of the test battery or composite test?

The theory which underlies aptitude testing provides an answer to the apparent dilemma for that particular type of test. For example, Anastasi (1982, p. 173) states:

For the prediction of practical criteria, not one but several tests may often be required. Most criteria are complex, the criterion measure depending on a number of different traits. A single test designed to measure such a criterion would thus have to be highly heterogeneous. ... however, a relatively homogeneous test, measuring largely a single trait, is more satisfactory because it yields less ambiguous scores. Hence, it is usually preferable to use a combination of several relatively homogeneous tests, each covering a different aspect of the criterion, rather than a single test consisting of a hodge-podge of many different kinds of items.

In other words, we should seek to maximize the internal consistency (that is, the reliability) of each component. The battery of tests so formed should aim to have maximum validity, defined principally as predictive validity. Concepts of the validity of a component or the reliability of a battery are of secondary importance.

In achievement testing, where validity cannot usually be established with reference to a criterion, the same principle of test construction is applied: each component should be made as reliable as possible. However, the correlations between the components are likely to be higher than is the case with aptitude tests; in the latter, as Anastasi (1982, p. 175) says, 'tests correlating highly with each other represent needless duplication'. In achievement tests, although the components represent facets of a complex attribute or curriculum, it is normally reasonable to expect at least modest correlation between components. If this is the case, the reliability of the test battery will be quite high usually (assuming that the components are reliable), since the sheer length of the test battery counts in favour of reliability.

Weighting

General considerations

Once the component scores are susceptible to being combined, consideration must be given to the weight each is to receive. In the case of aptitude tests, this is essentially an empirical matter. Consideration is given to the way in which the most accurate prediction of a criterion may be made, by means of the multiple regression technique introduced earlier; the regression weights obtained when the multiple regression equation is solved provide the weights for each component of the aptitude test battery. The components, combined with those weights applied, provide the best prediction of the criterion. Because this is readily understood as a concept, and because the mechanisms are discussed in most textbooks on educational or psychological measurement, no further consideration will be given to weighting in aptitude tests.

The weighting of the components of an achievement test is a technical matter which has received much attention from specialists. Here the intention is simply to present some of the issues and to provide references for more detailed reading. A comprehensive review of weighting is found in Wang and Stanley (1970). This needs to be complemented by more recent work.

The following discussion is of particular relevance to examinations in which the overall result is determined only by the aggregate mark and where the goal is to rank candidates on this aggregate. Such examinations are often referred to as 'norm-referenced' or 'peer-referenced'. If, as is more usual, a cutting score is set to represent minimum competence in each component or in the examination as a whole, then the issue of the contribution of a component to overall variance may be considered – as was suggested for aptitude testing – only for the wider perspective it provides.

As discussed above, an achievement test constitutes a definition of a subject by the choice of the components to be included in the final assessment. It is hoped that specialists in different situations and, to some extent, at different times will not disagree greatly on the choice of components. A comparison of examinations designed to be taken by family doctors at a comparable stage in training, for example, reveals a broad agreement on what should be tested. It is more likely that differences will arise over the relative importance of the components, reflecting slightly different circumstances, different purposes of the examination, and different attitudes among those empowered to make these essentially arbitrary decisions.

Planned and achieved weights

The decisions which are taken will be referred to as the planned weights of a battery of components. These may be expressed as percentages: for example, Paper 1, 20%; Paper 2, 30%; Oral, 25%; Clinical, 25%. In operational terms, these weights may be reflected directly in the maximum marks available for each component; using the same example, these might be respectively 80, 120, 100 and 100. Another simple approach would be to let 100 be the maximum mark for all four components, but, once marking is completed, to multiply Paper 1 marks by 0.8 and Paper 2 marks by 1.2 before adding in the marks on the other components.

Typically, discussions of weighting begin by demonstrating that the maximum mark of a component may bear little relationship to the actual impact which that component makes on the total score and hence on the final rank ordering of candidates. French (1981) provides such an example for a two-component examination (see Table 10.1). Paper 1 and Paper 2 are both marked out of a possible total of 100 and are intended to be of equal importance. A rank-order is established by Paper 1; it is completely reversed by Paper 2. When the two are combined, it is the rank-order of Paper 2 which is reflected in the final results, rather than

Table 10.1. *Example to show the lack of impact of maximum score on combined score*

Candidate	Paper 1	Rank	Paper 2	Rank	Total	Rank
A	30	4	95	1	125	1
B	50	3	74	2	124	2
C	60	2	61	3	121	3
D	70	1	50	4	120	4

Adapted from French (1981), with the permission of the British Psychological Society.

that of Paper 1 or some combination of the two. Paper 2 seems to be more important than Paper 1 – indeed, the final rank-order would have been the same if Paper 1 had not existed – and yet the two are intended to be of equal importance. In this example, since no effort is made to control the effective weights, the components have what are termed natural weights (Wang & Stanley, 1970).

The purpose of examples such as this is to introduce the discrepancy between the planned weight and what is termed the achieved weight. The former is a result of decisions taken before the examination; the latter is the reality of the candidates' performance. The research effort has been to reveal this discrepancy to decision-makers and to find ways of eliminating it.

Once it is realized that setting a maximum mark to reflect the planned weight does not guarantee correspondence with the achieved weight, it is usually the spread of marks that receives attention. A particularly striking case is the combination of scores on a multiple-choice test with those on an essay test using the system known as 'close marking'. An example of the problem has been described by Ashby & Baron (1986). There, essays were scored such that a mark of 50% indicated a bare pass, while 40% indicated 'appalling fail' and 60% 'superb pass'. If, as the authors imply, the range of possible marks is only 20, then the standard deviation is likely to be in the order of 4%, while a multiple-choice examination will aim normally at a standard deviation of 10%–15%. Combination of the two, without some adjustment of the scores, would clearly lead to the essay marks having a relatively small impact upon the resulting total score.

We are attempting, with achieved weights, to discover to what extent each component 'explains' or is responsible for the final rank-order or spread of candidates' marks. Mathematically, we seek the contribution of each component to the total variance. It is clear that if there is no variance on the scores on one component (i.e. all candidates get the same mark), that component will have no impact upon the rank-ordering derived by summing scores on the other components, since the effect is to add an equal amount to the score of each candidate. It may seem as though the greater the variance of a component, the greater is its effect upon the total variance.

If this were the case, then the obvious way to weight components so that the achieved weight was the same as the planned weight would be to intervene after the marking is complete and to constrain the variance of each component to reflect the planned weight. The standard deviation (which is the square root of the variance) of all components could be made equal, or could be set to reflect the ratio of differing weights in each component. The transformation of scores to allow for the standard deviation to be determined, rather than to arise as a chance feature of the candidates' responses or the scoring of them, is known as 'standardization'. Mathematically, it involves subtracting each 'raw' score from the mean of the raw scores, dividing by the standard deviation of the raw scores, and then multiplying the result by the desired standard deviation to arrive at a 'standard' score. The addition of a constant to each standard score is common (it avoids having to use negative numbers) and of course has the consequence that the transformed scores have a different mean as well as a different standard deviation; however, this is a secondary effect, since changing the mean has no impact upon the contribution of the component to the total score variance.

The previous paragraph began 'If this were the case'; unfortunately for those who practise the standardization of scores, it is not. The variance of the whole is not the same as the variance of the sum of the parts. Actually, the variance of the total score in a battery of tests is the sum of the variance of each component and of the covariance between the components. Covariance is a term used widely in the discussions of weighting. It is related to the coefficient of correlation and that more familiar term will be used here. Because of the need to take account of the inter-relationship of the components, the contribution of a component to the total needs to be defined as the standard deviation of that component divided by the standard deviation of the total score, the result to be multiplied by the coefficient of correlation between the component and the total. Therefore, a component which has quite a large standard deviation may nevertheless make a small contribution to the total variance because of the weak relationship between the two (Fowles, 1974; Adams & Murphy, 1982).

The standardization of component scores as discussed above does not change the relationships among them. In other words, the attempt to control the achieved weights by the use of standardized scores is only a partial solution because it fails to take account of the correlation coefficient. The practical importance of all this depends entirely on the nature of the test battery. If, for example, the correlation between all the components is similar and large, the use of standardized scores will be quite effective, because the influence of the term which is left out will be small. Terwilliger & Anderson (1969, p. 152) concluded from the data they analysed that 'standardizing component scores before computing a composite frequently results in only trivial changes from what would have been obtained by using the same nominal (i.e. planned) weights with raw scores'; Fowles (1974), using data from a quite different situation, was less pessimistic about the use of standardized scores.

However, if the above definition of contribution to total variance is accepted, what is required is a method of adjusting scores such that the achieved weights are equal to the planned weights, and one which takes account of both the standard deviation and the correlation. Such a method is offered in Adams & Wilmut (1982), to which, because of the complexity of the explanation, the interested reader may be referred.

The scaling of scores to harmonize planned and achieved weights is potentially a theoretical rather than a practical concern. Suppose, for example, three components of a test battery have the planned weights (in percentage terms) of 50, 20 and 30, and the achieved weights of 47.4, 20.7 and 31.9 (the example is from Fowles (1974)). Do we believe that those who determined the a priori weights did so with such accuracy that deviations of this order are significant or worth correcting? The responsibility of the examination authorities is to be aware of achieved weights and the possible discrepancy with planned weights, but not necessarily to eliminate very small discrepancies.

The goal of reliability can also determine the weighting of components. That is to say, components can be weighted in such a way as to maximize the reliability of the battery. There may be an attraction in including a component which is seen to be vital to a teaching programme (bearing in mind the ability of an examination to influence what is taught) but in minimizing the contribution of that component to the total because of the difficulty of assessing it reliably. Although this approach to weighting has been advocated by some authorities it is of doubtful value. As Newbould (1982) points out 'the main disadvantage of the technique is that, because the function being maximized is typically "flat", the resultant maximum is little higher than the composite reliability given by a quite different vector of component weights'.

Impact on candidates

By way of conclusion, we consider the extent to which combining components of assessment may influence the behaviour of candidates in an examination and, as a related point, how much an examination board should disclose of its procedures.

In achievement tests, the relative importance of components is usually made known to candidates and teachers in a syllabus or prospectus, and has the function of declaring how much emphasis should be given to each element of a course of study. Examinations often influence the curriculum overtly in this way. Even if the examining authority does not have this as an aim, it should disclose the relative importance of components and, if necessary, the procedures used to ensure that planned and achieved weights are harmonized (or, at least, monitored).

Probably of more importance to candidates' behaviour in the examination itself is knowledge of what has been described above as the 'pass/fail rules'. For example, if candidates believe that the examination model is a conjunctive one, in which it is necessary to demonstrate minimum competence in each component, they are likely to take a cautious approach to the assessment tasks – most obviously, to multiple-choice papers with penalty scoring. Such candidates would be at a clear disadvantage if the model were in fact a compensatory one, in which it is in their interests to maximize their scores on all components, in case excellence in one component is needed to offset mediocrity in another. The rules governing the combination of components in respect of pass/fail decisions should therefore be made clear, as should any requirement to demonstrate minimum competence in particular components.

References

Adams, R. & Murphy, R. J. L. (1982). The achieved weights of examination components. *Educational Studies*, **8**, 15–22.

Adams, R. & Wilmut, J. (1982). A measure of the weights of examination components, and scaling to adjust them. *The Statistician*, **30**, 263–9.

Anastasi, A. (1982). *Psychological Testing*. Fifth edition. New York: Macmillan.

Ashby, D. & Baron, D. N. (1986). Harmonizing multiple choice question marks with essay marks. *Medical Education*, **20**, 321–3.

Fowles, D. (1974). *CSE: two research studies.* Schools Council Examinations Bulletin *28.* London: Evans/Methuen.

French, S. (1981). Measurement theory and examinations. *British Journal of Mathematical and Statistical Psychology,* **34,** 38–49.

Guilford, J. P. & Fruchter, B. (1986). *Fundamental Statistics in Psychology and Education.* Sixth edition. New York: McGraw-Hill.

Newbould, C. A. (1982). 'Weighting examining components – a comparison of methods'. Paper presented at the Eighth Annual Conference of the British Educational Research Association.

Terwilliger, J. S. & Anderson, D. H. (1969). An empirical study of the effects of standardizing scores in the formation of linear composites, *Journal of Educational Measurement,* **6,** 145–154.

Torgerson, W. S. (1958). *Theory and Methods of Scaling.* New York: John Wiley & Sons.

Wang, N. W. & Stanley, J. C. (1970). Differential weighting: a review of methods and empirical studies. *Review of Educational Research,* **40,** 663–705.

11

In-training assessment

GRAHAME FELETTI (Editor), DONALD
CAMERON, BETH DAWSON-SAUNDERS,
JEAN-PIERRE des GROSEILLIERS, BRENDAN
DOOLEY, ELIZABETH FARMER and PAULINE
McAVOY

Fifty years ago, in British Dominion and North American medical institutions, certification of competence was based mainly on a final examination consisting of written essays and oral examinations. The objectives and scoring were implicit in, and subject to, the recognized expertise of the examiners. Not surprisingly, there was considerable variability in the standards of such examinations. Since then a whole new technology (the psychometrics) of educational assessment has emerged, aimed at improving the reliability and validity of examinations (see Chapter 8). This has been achieved largely by:

(i) Devising more 'objective' test instruments and formats (e.g. objective structured clinical examinations (OSCE), multiple-choice questions, standardized patients)
(ii) Defining more explicit examination objectives
(iii) Revising and reusing items pooled in data banks
(iv) Developing more universal procedures for determining pass/fail criteria

The final examination

In the last decade in particular, the final examination has become a formidable and omnibus approach to certification. Its advantages are highlighted in Table 11.1. Today's technology, evolving from application of psychometric theories, can confidently recommend minimum numbers of assessment items to attain pre-set levels of test reliability. It can also

151

Table 11.1. *Advantages and disadvantages of final examinations and in-training assessment*

Final examinations	In-training assessments
Advantages	
Measure what trainees *know*	Measure what trainees *do*
Possess high reliability	Possess high face validity
Are standardized across examinees	Can assess multiple attributes
Test-development methods are known	Can assess many attributes
Permit broad sampling of content	Can assess performance over time
Are efficient to administer	Use wider range of observers
Are efficient to score	Allow constructive feedback
Promote unbiased scoring	Are not time-constrained
Standard-setting methods are developed	Patients readily available
Psychometric methods are available	Inform trainers about training
	Non-invasive kind of assessment
Disadvantages	
Can assess limited attributes	May have low reliability
May influence trainee activities unduly	Not standardized across institutions
Time, cost, labour intensive	Not standardized across trainees
	Limited instruments available
	Training in assessment techniques is necessary
	Have potential for bias
	Require good record keeping
	Mix teacher and assessor functions

indicate: the trade-off in reliability when testing different skills separately or in combination; the optimal number of observers; or the best assessment procedure, instruments or response format which can lead to effective decisions on clinical competence.

Great strides have been made in improving the reliability and, to a lesser extent, the validity of performance on examinations. But in practical terms such recommendations can pose substantial logistical difficulties for certification, particularly when examinations must be conducted within a short period, at numerous locations, and for large numbers of candidates. Another major drawback is the substantial testing time, organizational effort and cost of running a comprehensive final examination. Lengthy examination periods for written tests may have been tolerable. However, the additional need for numerous OSCE stations or simulated patient encounters to give a reliable index of candidates' clinical (practical) skills now makes the whole process rather unwieldy and exhausting rather than exhaustive. Serious attention has been given to reducing this burden of assessment (see Bender *et al.*, 1990) including recommendations on the optimal number of observers or raters, the nature of clinical skills to be rated simultaneously and even the use of sequential testing (see Chapter 6).

Because of such problems, the role of the comprehensive final examination in the process of certification may need rethinking. Clearly it has a major impact on decision making, but why does it have such status? One reason may be an unwillingness to rely on assessments made during clinical attachments which studies show repeatedly to lack consistency and to fail to provide frequent observations of performance or effective feedback to students and residents (Abeykoon, 1983; Stillman *et al.*, 1987; Badesch *et al.*, 1989; Hall & Cotsonis, 1990). The requirement for better in-training assessment is clear but there is also a need for alternative approaches and more appropriate methods of assessment. Such approaches should be complementary to other forms of assessment such as examinations.

In-training assessment

In-training assessment (ITA) is defined here as systematic observation and feedback on habitual performance of candidates in real clinical settings during their training period. As highlighted in Table 11.1 its validity is strengthened by observations of interaction with actual patients in real time, using a wider range of observers than could be engineered for a comprehensive final examination.

Particular strengths of ITA evolve from the ability to observe and to assess trainees' behaviour regularly in many essential areas of clinical performance; skills which may be difficult or impossible to assess in an examination setting. These area include: procedural skills; interpersonal and communication skills; humanistic and professional attitudes to patients and families; application of socio-cultural knowledge and bio-ethics to health care; critical appraisal and self-directed learning skills; ability to work in teams of different kinds; and crisis and practice management skills.

In this context, different observers have the chance to evaluate the performance of each graduate in these areas as they progress through vocational training. The observers may be peers or other health professionals, practice staff and patients. Systematic collection of assessments from them would build up a comprehensive picture of the doctor's performance and should also improve the quality of assessment by helping to reduce observer or instrument bias. This information, about a candidate's clinical competence across situations and observers, may give not only more robust measurement of their skills, but also a more valid prediction of their habitual professional behaviour.

ITA seems equally appropriate for making competency decisions about undergraduates, postgraduates and even foreign medical graduates whose performance may need frequent observation or assessment soon after their acceptance into certain programmes. If ITA takes place in the practice setting, where habitual behaviour of the doctor is easier to detect, it enables integrated assessment of entire clinical tasks to be made. This approach also appears to be a more collegial or educational activity, allowing timely and specific feedback about performance to be given to the trainee. In addition, ITA may not rely so heavily on the stricter requirements needed for a final examination.

There is a growing realization that ITA can provide meaningful data as part of the assessment process for certification of competence, evidenced by a number of recent studies. Two issues seem to be important. First, the instruments used may be identical with those adopted for final examination. Incorporating them in ITA at the very least reduces the strain of such assessment on all concerned, and enhances its educational value to candidates. But ITA should not be confused with formative assessment; the latter simply being 'learning experiences' which do not count for or against a candidate's progress in any formal sense. Nor is ITA just a premature, site-specific alternative to running a comprehensive final examination. Its real strength lies in the balance, timing and nature of the situations used to test clinical competencies.

The second issue seems to be the kind of data provided by some instruments and in particular their 'subjectivity' or lack of traditional reliability. Measures of multiple-rater agreement, for example, were not well defined or 'user friendly' until recently. Organizations such as the American Board of Internal Medicine (ABIM) and Royal College of Physicians and Surgeons of Canada set good examples. The latter makes explicit the criteria to be used in their final in-training evaluation report (FITER), and gives clear instructions on how best to use this form of assessment.

The following examples review briefly some of the more common methods used for investigating ITA, enabling us to see how research is proceeding and what seems necessary to improve the acceptability of ITA for certification. First, however, two approaches used in medicine to define the content of clinical training are described.

Determining the content of training

Critical incident technique

This widely-accepted technique of job or task analysis from personnel training may be applied to training programmes in medicine. Such an approach was used many years ago to identify categories of competence for the internship (Hubbard *et al.*, 1965) and the practice of internal medicine (Sanazaro & Williamson, 1968). More recently this technique has been used to determine categories of behaviour in obstetrics and gynaecology residency training (Altmaier *et al.*, 1988), in radiology training at three separate institutions (Altmaier *et al.*, 1989), and in paediatrics training (Altmaier *et al.*, 1990). The critical-incident methodology has also been used successfully to determine the major problems faced by pre-registration house officers (interns) (Calman & Donaldson, 1991). Once the categories are determined, measures can be developed to assess the behaviours.

Surveys

Surveys and related techniques may be used to determine perceived importance of content as well as the content itself (Dawson-Saunders *et al.*, 1990). A survey of all USA internal medicine training programme directors was used to obtain opinions regarding which procedural skills residents should master during training and the number of procedures they need to complete in order to develop and to maintain their skills (Wigton *et al.*, 1989).

Methods of assessment

Great efforts have been made in recent years to apply the rigour of standardization expected in examinations to the in-training situation.

In-training written examinations

Based on the performance of all examinees, in-training written examinations were found to have predictive validity for performance on a certification examination in family medicine (Leigh *et al.*, 1990). Performance of all residents on a pathology residency programme in-training examination discriminated among levels of residency training, although the differences were less than expected (Lockard *et al.*, 1985).

Standardized techniques other than written examinations

General

A study of methods used to teach and to assess clinical skills of Australian family medicine trainees in practice settings showed a preference for case review and an avoidance of direct observation (Farmer & Taylor, 1990). An ABIM survey of all first-time takers of the 1988 certifying examination in internal medicine was undertaken to learn what methods were being used to assess residents' clinical skills (Day *et al.*, 1990). The methods most often used were medical record audit (51%), the in-training examination (52%) and training in advanced cardiac support (92%). Eighty-three per cent of residents had undergone a structured clinical examination exercise (CEX) developed by the ABIM in which initially the resident was observed performing a physical examination and then had to present the findings and a plan of management. However, only 32% had undergone two or more CEXs. Other than their CEX, 55% and 36% respectively had never had their history-taking skills or physical examination techniques observed directly during their training. In another study of the CEX, faculty internists at one hospital differed in their observations of residents and were found to document little, suggesting the need to provide faculty assessors with training as observers (Herbers *et al.*, 1989).

In a predictive validity study, residents from training programmes that provide extensive, well-supervised educational experiences in ambulatory care had higher scores on the certifying examination in internal medicine (Norcini *et al.*, 1987*a*).

Assessments by faculty supervisors

The ABIM requires programme directors to rate residents in overall clinical competence and its essential components on a scale from 1 to 9; ratings were correlated moderately with performance on the certification examination over a five-year period (Norcini *et al.*, 1987*b*).

A confidential system to assess professional progress every six months has been used in an anaesthesiology residency programme (Jago, 1989). A method to quantify daily supervisor comments has been reported to improve feedback turn-around time to increase the breadth of evaluators and settings, and to improve documentation (Rhoton, 1990).

Faculty supervisors with more years' experience as preceptors were better able to predict resident's cognitive levels than those with limited experience in three family practice training programmes. The authors suggested that inability to assess accurately may influence the teacher–resident relationship negatively (Taylor & Lipsky, 1990).

Self assessments

A comparison of self and supervisor ratings of first-year residents graduating from one medical school found evidence that self ratings were more sensitive to specific areas of strength and weakness while supervisor ratings tended to be more global in nature (Kolm & Verhulst, 1987).

Oral examination

A structured oral examination in a surgical residency training programme was found to have psychometric properties exceeding those of traditional oral examinations (Anastakis *et al.*, 1991). Annual in-training oral examinations in paediatrics identified 'problem' residents at one institution better than by using only their scores on written in-training examinations (Quattlebaum, *et al.*, 1988).

Consultation reports

A preliminary study using outpatient consultation letters from senior students and junior resident staff to assess problem definition, investigation and management skills in two clinical services had promising results (McCain *et al.*, 1988).

Assessment of humanistic skills

A form designed to be used by nurses to assess the humanistic behaviour of residents was found to provide reliable assessments in general medicine, cardiology and haematology-oncology (Butterfield *et al.*, 1987). A follow-up study found that five or six nurses were needed to provide reliable ratings and that the information was somewhat different from that provided by medical staff (Butterfield & Mazzaferri, 1991). Another study, comparing nurse and doctor ratings of internal medicine residents in two hospitals, found the ratings to be correlated only moderately with the doctors being more lenient raters than the nurses (Kaplan & Centor, 1990).

Psychological studies

Surveys of emotions and attitudes of two classes of internal medicine residents found relationships among their psychological states and their clinical performance (Girard & Hickam, 1991).

Ratings by peers

Global ratings by professional associates of nine aspects of clinical competence were reported to be reliable and to have the potential to identify physicians with low performance (Ramsey *et al.*, 1989); 10 to 20 ratings were needed for reliable estimates (Carline *et al.*, 1989). Ratings of surgery resident performance by peers in one programme were highly correlated with ratings by supervisors (Risucci *et al.*, 1989). Assessment of emergency medicine residents by nurses in one hospital was reported as having positive consequences on resident behaviour (Tintinalli, 1989). The critical incident technique has been suggested as another approach to collecting data on actual clinical performance (Newble, 1983).

Ratings by patients

Research at the ABIM on patient satisfaction questionnaires indicated that ratings from 30 to 50 patients were required to give stable estimates of individual practitioners (Swanson *et al.*, 1990).

Standardized patients

Standardized patients provide an increasingly popular way to obtain assessment of a range of clinical skills (see Chapter 6; Barrows, 1987). A comprehensive review of the literature has been published by van der Vleuten & Swanson (1990; see Chapter 8), including the number of standardized patient problems needed for reliable assessment. Research in several settings has indicated that junior doctors are unable to distinguish between actual and standardized patients when they are encountered in an everyday setting (Gordon *et al.*, 1988). In a study of residents from 19 training programmes, Stillman and colleagues (1991) concluded that standardized patients were best used to assess data gathering and interviewing skills and suggested that standardized patient scores may be measuring something different from other assessment methods. A system of videotaping interns' interviews with standardized patients has been used to provide educational feedback to interns regarding the quality of their history and physical examination (Edelstein & Ruder, 1990) and to assess a variety of other skills, such as giving advice to the patient on prevention (Gordon *et al.*, 1989; Hoppe *et al.*, 1990).

Objective structured clinical examination

Scores on an OSCE that included standardized patient stations at one institution discriminated between the performance of paediatrics residents at various levels of training (demonstrating construct validity) better than either in-training examination scores or performance ratings (Joorabchi, 1991). OSCE scores for a group of residents in internal medicine did not correlate well with overall faculty ratings of clinical performance and correlated only moderately with scores on the certification examination (Petrusa *et al.*, 1990). Performance by foreign medical graduates on an OSCE was found to predict their performance in an internship preparation programme at five medical schools (Rothman *et al.*, 1990).

Bias

One of the most difficult problems in in-training assessment is the elimination of bias (see also Chapter 6). A review of 19 years of evaluations in one surgical residency training programme found that average ratings for a sample of male and female residents were nearly the same, regardless of whether they came from male or female faculty (Hayward *et al.*, 1987). In assessment of humanistic skills, Kaplan & Centor (1990) found that nurse ratings of internal medical residents varied by gender of resident and type of nursing unit. Male and female patients in one hospital were found to differ in the behaviours they valued in interns, with female patients placing more importance than male patients on personal manner and concern (Lieberman *et al.*, 1989). Older patients and whites at two hospitals were more satisfied with the performance of their interns, while college-educated, employed, male patients were less satisfied (Matthews *et al.*, 1987). Patient attitudes at one institution were said to be influenced by the personal appearance of doctors; however, patient attitudes were less affected than those of other doctors (Gjerdingen *et al.*, 1987). A study of family medicine physicians at one institution found a greater effect of age and style of dress than gender on patient attitudes (McNaughton-Filion *et al.*, 1991).

Table 11.2. *Models of certification*

Model 1: Certification based only on a final examination, with ITA playing no formal part
Model 2: Certification determined exclusively by ITA without a final examination
Model 3: A satisfactory standard based on ITA must be attained before candidates can sit the final examination
Model 4: In addition to reaching a satisfactory standard in order to sit the final examination, ITA performance influences or forms part of the decision-making process for certification
Model 5: All candidates allowed to sit the final examination, but ITA performance contributes directly to the decision for certification

Models of certification

Five alternative models for certifying clinical competence may be advanced (see Table 11.2). Each has advantages and disadvantages.

Model 1: The final exam is all that counts!

The relative advantages and disadvantages of this approach have been summarized in Table 11.1. Reliance on performance in any final examination effectively ignores the earlier-cited research evidence accumulated from various sources highlighting the wide range of clinical experiences during the training programme. As Miller (1990) points out, this approach overlooks major differences between what candidates *do* (their habitual behaviour) and what they *can do* (their examination behaviour). Norman (1990) is analysing what facets of clinical competence are observed better in naturalistic settings than under examination conditions. But we should be wary of attempts to 'build in' examination items (stations) to assess these less tangible or more 'natural' competencies.

One other point can be made about certification by final examination. Current difficulties in the supervision of residency candidates in natural settings has already been raised as one justification for the block testing of clinical skills components (e.g. history taking, physical examination, communication) in final examinations. By their very nature, and the large number of observations recommended for reliable estimations of such competencies, these assessments seem to be tested far more appropriately in the training period itself.

Model 2: In-training assessment will sort them out!

Such an approach may appeal initially to candidates (weary of the annual ritual of examination 'performance', particularly the three-day triathlons of written, oral and clinical tests). But there are several important and unjustifiable assumptions in this model. First, that candidates can deal successfully with everyday clinical encounters in their training period; second, that the kind of clinical experiences at their given training site offer sufficient opportunity for developing the required competencies; and third, that their behaviour can be monitored systematically and fairly, resulting in an informed, clear and objective judgement of competence.

Model 3: In-training assessment: a preliminary step towards final examination

This approach uses in-training assessment as a basic screening of candidates for the final examination. It implies that the rating of candidates' competence in the real practice situation is important (to the certifying body) and that candidates and supervisors alike will need to be clear on the stated objectives, the ways and times these will be assessed, and the likely avenues for effective feedback and remediation.

This process is probably the most flexible, and potentially the most collegial in terms of the tutor/assessor role of the supervisor. However, it has some tender spots. For example, it may suffer from interpersonal conflict or unclear expectations between candidate and supervisor. Simple procedural safeguards need stating and reinforcing to candidates and examiners alike. The way in which performance on ITA is prerequisite to the final examination must also be clear.

Draft guidelines by the Royal College of Physicians and Surgeons of Canada on its in-training evaluation and the FITER take up the challenge of overcoming many previous concerns. For example, that College expects each specialty or subspecialty to develop its own FITER, in keeping with its own programme objectives. It focuses attention on the residents' performance in the final period of training, and is not to be calculated as an average of earlier reports. The FITER aims to represent the consensus of an appropriate group of faculty who have observed the resident on numerous occasions. The resident is expected to be told of the process at the earliest opportunity and the procedure is to be implemented from the start of the training period. Clear statements are also made in the draft on using criteria and rating categories and how best to incorporate ITA results in decision-making (e.g. upgrading otherwise borderline final examination performance).

Models 4 and 5: In-training assessment directly contributes to the certification decision but in different ways

Adopting these models clearly requires the provision of consistent information about candidates' habitual behaviour in clinical settings on carefully defined components of competence. For example, ratings from a range of observers over a well-defined period will help to provide representative, unbiased indices of clinical competence. Such an approach must distinguish clearly between formative and summative ratings. However, it could also include inherently more reliable assessments using standardized patients, OSCEs, and short written tests conducted at the training site.

For Model 4, an overall satisfactory rating on ITA may be used to compensate for a marginal final examination performance. With Model 5, the ITA may have two status levels. At the stronger level it is taken as an essential hurdle which, like the final examination, must be completed satisfactorily before certification. At the lower level, overall ITA score is weighted (e.g. 50%) and then added to the final examination score. From this distribution of total scores a 'passing mark' for certification can be decided.

These two models have their limitations. Model 4 allows compensation for poor performance (e.g. on knowledge, critical thinking, research skills) in the final examination by having a high overall performance on ITA. With Model 5, difficulties may arise in processing candidates whose results are not satisfactory on ITA but who still pass the final examination. Several ways of addressing these technical difficulties in combining components of assessment are discussed in Chapter 10.

Conclusion

This chapter has attempted to identify acceptable alternatives to the final examination model of certification on the basis that this approach is becoming too labour-intensive, fails to assess validly some important clinical skills and professional behaviours, and is not educationally sound for medical training programmes of 2 to 4 years' duration. An alternative approach is to use in-training assessment, but probably in conjunction with final examinations. The choice of model will depend on various factors, including: the resources available for in-training assessment; confidence in the programme and quality of the trainees; and the willingness of the certifying body to accept less reliable, but potentially more valid, indices in reaching their decisions about candidates. What has not yet been addressed, either here or in the current research literature, is how to train faculty and other health professionals to implement in-training assessment effectively and fairly.

References

Abeykoon, P. (1983). An evaluation of training in family health for medical students and interns in Sri Lanka. *Medical Education*, **17**, 240–6.

Altmaier, E. M., Johnson, S. R., Tarico, V. S. & Laube, D. (1988). An empirical specification of residency performance dimensions. *Obstetrics and Gynecology*, **72**, 126–30.

Altmaier, E. M., McGuinness, G., Wood, P., Ross, P. R., Bartley, J. & Smith, W. (1990). Defining successful performance among pediatric residents. *Pediatrics*, **85**, 139–43.

Altmaier, E., Smith, W. L., Wood, P., Ross, R., Montgomery, W. J., Klattee, E., Imray, T., Shields, J. & Frankien, E. A., Jr (1989). Cross-institutional stability of behavioral criteria desirable for success in radiology residency. *Investigative Radiology*, **24**, 249–51.

Anastakis, D. J., Cohen, R. & Reznick, R. K. (1991). The structured oral examination as a method for assessing surgical residents. *American Journal of Surgery*, **162**, 67–70.

Badesch, D. B., McClellan, M. D., Wheeler, A. P., Archer, P. G., Schwarz, M. I. & Petty, T. L. (1989). A model for the objective assessment of clinical training programs: the initial application of two pulmonary medicine fellowship programs. *American Review of Respiratory Diseases*, **140**, 1136–42.

Barrows, H. (1987). *Simulated (Standardized) Patients and Other Human Simulations*. Chapel Hill: Health Sciences Consortium.

Bender, W., Hiemstra, R. J., Scherpbier, A. J. J. A. & Zwierstra, R. P. (Eds.) (1990). *Teaching and Assessing Clinical Competence*. Groningen: BoekWerk Publications.

Butterfield, P. S. & Mazzaferri, E. L. (1991). A new rating form for use by nurses in assessing residents' humanistic behavior. *Journal of General Internal Medicine*, **6**, 155–61.

Butterfield, P. S., Mazzaferri, E. L. & Sachs, L. A. (1987). Nurses as evaluators of the humanistic behavior of internal medicine residents. *Journal of Medical Education*, **62**, 842–9.

Calman, K. C. & Donaldson, M. (1991). The pre-registration house officer year: a critical incident study. *Medical Education*, **25**, 51–9.

Carline, J. D., Wenrich, M. & Ramsey, P. G. (1989). Characteristics of ratings of physician competence by professional associates. *Evaluation in the Health Professions*, **12**, 409–23.

Dawson-Saunders, B., Feltovich, P. J., Coulson, R. L. & Steward, D. E. (1990). A survey of medical school teachers to identify basic biomedical concepts medical students should understand. *Academic Medicine*, **65**, 448–54.

Day, S. C., Grosso, L. J., Norcini, J. J., Jr, Blank, L. L., Swanson, D. B. & Horne, M. H. (1990). Residents' perception of evaluation procedures used by their training program. *Journal of General Internal Medicine*, **5**, 421–6.

Edelstein, D. R. & Ruder, H. J. (1990). Assessment of clinical skills using videotapes of the complete medical interview and physical examination. *Medical Teacher*, **12**, 155–62.

Farmer, E. A. & Taylor, S. (1990). Assessment of teaching by Family Medicine Programme vocational trainees. *Australian Family Physician*, **19**, 549–57.

Girard, D. E. & Hickam, D. H. (1991). Predictors of clinical performance among internal medicine residents. *Journal of General Internal Medicine*, **6**, 150–4.

Gjerdingen, D. J., Simpson, D. E. & Titus, S. L. (1987). Patients' and physicians' attitudes regarding the physician's professional appearance. *Archives of Internal Medicine*, **147**, 1209–12.

Gordon, J., Sanson-Fisher, R. & Saunders, N. A. (1988). Identification of simulated patients by interns in a casualty setting. *Medical Education*, **22**, 533–8.

Gordon, J., Saunders, N. A. & Sanson-Fisher, R. W. (1989). Evaluating interns' performance using simulated patients in a casualty department. *Medical Journal of Australia*, **151**, 18–21.

Hall, J. R. & Cotsonis, G. A. (1990). Analysis of residents' performances on the In-Training Examination of the American Board of Anesthesiology–American Society of Anesthesiologists. *Academic Medicine*, **65**, 475–7.

Hayward, C. Z., Sachdeva, A. & Clarke, J. R. (1987). Is there gender bias in the evaluation of surgical residents? *Surgery*, **102**, 297–9.

Herbers, J. E., Jr, Noel, G. L., Cooper, G. S., Harvey, J., Pangaro, L. N. & Weaver, M. J. (1989). How accurate are faculty evaluations of clinical competence? *Journal of General Internal Medicine*, **4**, 202–8.

Hoppe, R. B., Farquhar, L. J., Henry, R. & Stoffelmayr, B. (1990). Residents' attitudes towards and skills in counseling: using undetected standardized patients. *Journal of General Internal Medicine*, **5**, 415–20.

Hubbard, J. P., Levit, E. H., Schumacher, C. F. & Schnabel, T. G. (1965). An objective evaluation of clinical competence. *New England Journal of Medicine*, **272**, 1321–8.

Jago, R. H. (1989). Confidential professional reports. A method of assessing the career progress and prospects of anaesthetic senior house officers. *Anaesthesia*, **44**, 153–6.

Joorabchi, B. (1991). Objective structured clinical examination in a pediatric residency program. *American Journal of Disorders in Children*, **145**, 757–62.

Kaplan, C. B. & Centor, R. M. (1990). The use of nurses to evaluate house officers' humanistic behavior. *Journal of General Internal Medicine*, **5**, 410–4.

Kolm, P. & Verhulst, S. J. (1987). Comparing self- and supervisor-evaluations: a different view. *Evaluation in the Health Professions*, **10**, 80–9.

Leigh, T. M., Johnson, T. P. & Pisacano, N. J. (1990). Predictive validity of the American Board of Family Practice In-Training Examination. *Academic Medicine*, **65**, 454–7.

Lieberman, P. B., Sledge, W. H. & Matthews, D. A. (1989). Effect of patient gender on evaluation of intern performance. *Archives of Internal Medicine*, **149**, 1825–9.

Lockard, W. T., Jr, Beeler, M. F., Stembridge, V. A. & Troy, L. A. (1985). First national in-service examination for pathology residents. *American Journal of Clinical Pathology*, **83**, 1–6.

Matthews, D. A., Sledge, W. H. & Lieberman, P. B. (1987). Evaluation of intern performance by medical inpatients. *American Journal of Medicine*, **83**, 938–44.

McCain, G. A., Molineux, J. E., Pederson, L. & Stuart, R. K. (1988). Consultation letters as a method for assessing in-training performance in a department of medicine. *Evaluation in the Health Professions*, **11**, 21–42.

McNaughton-Filion, L., Chen, J. S. & Norton, P. G. (1991). The physician's appearance. *Family Medicine*, **23**, 208–11.

Miller, G. E. (1990). The assessment of clinical skill/competence/performance. *Academic Medicine*, **65**, S63–67.

Newble, D. I. (1983). The critical incident technique: a new approach to the assessment of clinical performance. *Medical Education*, **17**, 401–3.

Norcini, J. J., Grosso, L. J., Shea, J. A. & Webster, G. D. (1987*a*). The relationship between features of residency training and ABIM certifying examination performance. *Journal of General Internal Medicine*, **2**, 330–6.

Norcini, J. J., Webster, G. D., Grosso, L. J., Blank, L. L. & Benson, J. A., Jr (1987*b*). Ratings of residents' clinical competence and performance on certification examination. *Journal of Medical Education*, **62**, 457–62.

Norman, G. R. (1990). Summary of the conference. In *Teaching and Assessing Clinical Competence,* ed. W. Bender, R. J. Hiemstra, A. J. J. A. Scherpbier & R. P. Zwierstra, pp. 599–609. Groningen: BoekWerk Publications.

Petrusa, E. R., Blackwell, T. A. & Ainsworth, M. A. (1990). Reliability and validity of an objective structured clinical examination for assessing the clinical performance of residents. *Archives of Internal Medicine*, **150**, 573–7.

Quattlebaum, T. G., Darden, P. M. & Sperry, J. B. (1988). Predicting resident clinical performance with in-training examinations. *Proceedings of the Annual Conference of Research in Medical Education*, **27**, 182–7.

Ramsey, P. G., Carline, J. D., Inui, T. S., Larson, E. B., LoGerfo, J. P. & Wenrich, M. D. (1989). Predictive validity of certification by the American Board of Internal Medicine. *Annals of Internal Medicine*, **110**, 719–26.

Rhoton, M. F. (1990). A new method to evaluate clinical performance and critical incidents in anaesthesia: quantification of daily comments by teachers. *Medical Education*, **24**, 280–9.

Risucci, D. A., Tortolani, A. J. & Ward, R. J. (1989). Ratings of surgical residents by self, supervisors and peers. *Surgery, Gynecology and Obstetrics*, **169**, 519–26.

Rothman, A. I., Cohen, R. & Ross, J. (1990). Evaluating the clinical skills of foreign medical school graduates participating in an internship preparation program. *Academic Medicine*, **65**, 391–5.

Sanazaro, P.J. & Williamson, J. W. (1968). A classification of physician performance in internal medicine. *Journal of Medical Education*, **43**, 389–97.

Stillman, P. L., Regan, M. B. & Swanson, D. B. (1987). A diagnostic fourth-year performance assessment. *Archives of Internal Medicine*, **147**, 1981–5.

Stillman, P., Swanson, D., Regan, M. B. *et al.* (1991). Assessment of clinical skills of residents utilizing standardized patients. A follow-up study and recommendations for application. *Annals of Internal Medicine*, **114**, 393–401.

Swanson, D. B., Webster, G. D. & Norcini, J. J. (1990). Precision of patient ratings of residents' humanistic qualities: how many items and patients are enough? In *Teaching and Assessing Clinical Competence*, ed. W. Bender, R. Hiemstra, A. J. J. A. Scherpbier & R. Zwierstra, pp. 423–31. Groningen: BoekWerk Publications.

Taylor, C. & Lipsky, M. S. (1990). A study of the ability of physician faculty members to predict resident performance. *Family Medicine*, **22**, 296–8.

Tintinalli, J. E. (1989). Evaluation of emergency medicine residents by nurses. *Academic Medicine*, **64**, 49–50.

van der Vleuten, C. & Swanson, D. (1990). Assessment of clinical skills with standardized patients: state of the art. *Teaching and Learning in Medicine*, **2**, 58–76.

Wigton, R. S., Blank, L. L., Nicolas, J. A. & Tape, T. G. (1989). Procedural skills training in internal medicine residencies. A survey of program directors. *Annals of Internal Medicine*, **111**, 932–8.

Part D

Recertification of clinical competence

12

Maintenance of competence and/or recertification: policy considerations

RAJA BANDARANAYAKE (Editor), DONALD
CAMERON, JEAN-PIERRE des GROSEILLIERS,
JACQUES des MARCHAIS, BARRIE McCANN
and CEES van der VLEUTEN

The focus of studies on medical education has tended to be on the undergraduate phase to a large extent, and on the postgraduate phase to a lesser extent. Yet the former occupies a relatively small period in the continuum of medical education. All the effort that is directed towards improving training in this phase, such as problem-based learning and orientation to the community, could be negated in a relatively short time in practice if efforts are not made towards maintaining the skills in the protracted period of continuing education.

This latter phase has been the focus of renewed interest in medical education recently. In 1990, in one region of the World Health Organization alone, three international activities had, as their theme, 'continuing medical education' (CME). Recertification is one important component of CME.

This chapter was developed from the discussions of a working group (at the Fifth Cambridge Conference) which was entrusted with the task of making policy recommendations with regard to the issue of recertification of the medical practitioner, irrespective of the specialty or sub-specialty engaged in by the latter. It describes two contrasting conceptual approaches to the issue of recertification, comparing their advantages and disadvantages. It also examines some issues relating to implementation and evaluation of the preferred approach.

Purposes of recertification

The basic purpose behind any recertification procedure is the maintenance of competence of the practitioner. Maintenance of competence is important for several reasons:

  (i) Accountability to the public who are entitled to the highest possible
       standards of medical care
 (ii) Accountability to the profession which insists that its standards are
       maintained in line with advances in that body of knowledge and
       skills which comprise the profession
(iii) Accountability to the body politic, usually at governmental level,
       which provides the funding for health care and in return expects the
       health personnel it employs to provide the highest quality of care
       within the limits of the available resources
 (iv) Legal accountability, demanded by the employer and insurance
       companies, to avoid litigation
  (v) The need to maintain the professional's skills *pari passu* with
       advancing technology
 (vi) To provide a baseline against which incompetence may be judged

This chapter argues that the primary purpose of any recertification
procedure should be the maintenance of competence of the majority of
the practitioners, rather than the identification of incompetence in the
minority who are at the lower end of the distribution of competence.
However, a spectrum of approaches was identified, ranging between the
two extremes of maintenance of competence, on the one hand, and
identification of incompetence, on the other. Approaches vary in the
extent to which these two purposes are served among different countries,
and among certifying bodies within a given country. The experiences in
countries of the members of the group are outlined below. However, it is
necessary first to clarify the meanings of some of the terms used in this
field, as some degree of confusion exists in the literature.

Terminology

'Certification' is a testimony to the fact that an individual has completed
an appropriate form of training. It can be of two types: certification of
attendance at a training course or courses and certification of competence. The former is related to the 'process' of training, while the latter
testifies to the 'product' of training as competent. In the medical profession a certificate of undergraduate or postgraduate training is usually
of the latter type. In the case of undergraduate education a certificate of
competence implies that the individual has completed a period of formal
training satisfactorily; in postgraduate certification this may not always be
so.

'Licensure', on the other hand, is defined as 'formal permission from a constituted authority to do something ... a certificate of permission' (Bowmer, 1991). As Bowmer points out, while 'certification (of competence) may be acceptable for licensure, they are unlikely to be equivalent'. For example, in many countries a period of approved apprenticeship is required for the newly certified medical graduate before a licencing body grants a licence to practise medicine. The right of licensure is usually vested in bodies which are entrusted by society to utilize the skills of the professional gained through training. Such bodies are often not the training institution itself. In most countries this function is performed by state or national health authorities.

'Recertification' is the process by which a professional body testifies intermittently to the competence of each of its members, either with or without a period of formal retraining. 'Relicensure', on the other hand, is the means by which an employing body grants permission to the practitioner, whose original licence to practise has lapsed for some reason, to continue or recommence practice. Logically, then, one can be recertified only if one is certified in the first instance (Silver, 1989). Recertification should, therefore, be the responsibility of the body that issued the certificate. In the absence of time-limited certification it is questionable whether a certificate, once issued, could be withdrawn. Thus any professional body which is considering the introduction of a system of recertification should first institute a system where the original certificate to practise is given for a limited period. For example, the Royal Australian College of Obstetricians and Gynaecologists (RACOG) incorporated in its constitution the notion of time-limited Fellowship at the time it was founded in 1978 (see Chapter 5). The American Board of Ophthalmology announced that all those who pass their examinations from 1992 onwards will be certified for a limited period only (Murchland, 1988). Currently, 16 of the 23 American Specialty Boards have introduced time-limited certification or are committed to do so, for periods ranging from seven to, most commonly, ten years (see Chapter 4). Langsley (1991) estimated that by 1994 more than 95% of American diplomates who receive general or subspecialty certificates will find that they expire within ten years.

Relicensure, however, is the prerogative of the licensing body, which has the power to withdraw the licence of any person who fails to satisfy the requirements for continuing licensure, whether related to incompetence, negligence or malpractice.

Practices in different countries

In Australia, the issue of recertification of the medical practitioner has surfaced several times, but no uniformity exists in the practices of the various bodies responsible for the continuing education of the professional. Only one of the specialist colleges (RACOG) has introduced a system of mandatory recertification. The system is dependent on the accumulation of a minimum number of 'cognate points' for participation in continuing medical education (CME) activities. The Royal Australian College of General Practitioners, while not insisting on mandatory recertification, expects its members to participate in professional development activities within a quality assurance programme, and indirectly contributes to a reregistration scheme of the federal government (see Chapter 5). Several other Colleges are actively developing their recertification schemes which are expected to be in place within the next two to three years. All are to be based on participation in CME but also include elements of audit and peer review.

In Canada there are two national certifying bodies (see also Chapter 4), the College of Family Physicians of Canada (CFPC) and the Royal College of Physicians and Surgeons of Canada (RCPSC). The latter certifies 43 specialties and subspecialties, and recognizes another nine subspecialties by way of accreditation without certification. It established a maintenance of competence (MOCOMP) pilot program in 1990 in collaboration with nine national specialty societies. The programme features voluntary enrolment, opportunity for selection of options, documentation of CME activities and confidential summaries of aggregate results. The pilot project will be subject to a two-year in-depth evaluation of impact on the practices of specialists. The CFPC has a maintenance of certification program in which all certificants are required to participate every five years. Maintenance of a defined standard of competence is seen as a shared responsibility between the College and the individual certificant. Members are also required to meet the College's study credit requirements on an annual basis. The maintenance of certification program is not an examination but a self-learning programme, based on multiple-choice questions, aimed at assisting the certificant in reviewing current knowledge of the primary care literature. Participation in the programme, rather than achieving a minimum score, is required to maintain status as a certificant.

In the Netherlands, no formal legislation regarding CME or recertification exists as the Government is reluctant to prescribe activities in the area of recertification. The professional community, consisting of several Colleges, strives for an internal quality assurance system, which is accredited externally by the authorities. Thus CME and recertification are the responsibility of the professional community. Recertification through formal processes such as examinations has not been considered, and the emphasis is on educational activities, such as courses, peer review and definition of quality and standards of care. For example, the Dutch College of General Practitioners initiated, through a study of the literature and discussion with practitioners, a process of defining and publishing standards of care. Subsequently, these are used in CME courses and in peer review procedures, as well as for test development and assessment. The latter is used purely for the purposes of screening (identifying areas of weakness in groups for laying down further educational policy) and of formative assessment (providing individual feedback for improvement).

A spectrum of approaches

The extremes of a spectrum of approaches to recertification have been alluded to above. At one end the focus is on the identification of incompetence, at the other on the maintenance of competence. Berwick (1989; see Chapter 5) referred to the former as the 'Theory of Bad Apples' and the latter as the 'Theory of Continuous Improvement'. Taking the analogy further, the former tries to identify the 'bad apples' and to remove them from the system, whereas the latter places emphasis on keeping the 'good apples', which are the majority, in optimal condition. Any strategy for recertification could be based on a philosophy which incorporated the desirable characteristics of each of these two extremes. The ideal strategy would focus primarily on maintaining the competence of all practitioners, yet would incorporate a system of identifying the minority who were not maintaining competence.

Table 12.1 lists key words describing each end of the spectrum of approaches. These characteristics do not each belong exclusively to the corresponding end of the spectrum, but tend, in general, to be associated with that particular end. For example, a system which focuses exclusively on identifying the minority who are 'poor performers' and who do not take the necessary steps to improve their performance tends to be imposed from above. It often depends on a system of examinations which are of a summative nature; is punitive rather than reward oriented; and is

Table 12.1. *Key words associated with the extremes of a
spectrum of approaches to recertification*

'Bad apples approach'	'Good apples approach'
Comprehensive	Specific
Teaching	Learning
Imposed	Self-directed
Content specified	Content determined by participant
Minority-based	Majority-based
Summative	Formative
Examinations	Participatory, on-going assessment
Punitive	Rewarding
Distrust of participants	Faith in participants

based on a lack of faith in the ability of the doctor to be responsible for
his/her own learning and assessment. On the other hand, a system which
focuses exclusively on maintaining and ensuring competence: is based on
faith in his/her ability to assume responsibility for learning; depends on
informal assessment of a formative nature with feedback to enable the
physician to correct deficiencies and to capitalize on strengths; and seeks
to reward rather than to punish. In the former approach, content of
learning and assessment is specified usually by authorities with a focus on
teaching; whereas in the latter it is determined by the participant with a
focus on learning. Thus, content tends to be comprehensive in the former
and more specific and targeted to individual needs in the latter.

There is evidence that neither of these extremes is likely to be effective
in raising the quality of care provided by the profession. Glassock *et al.*
(1991) report that previous attempts by the American Board of Internal
Medicine to mount voluntary recertification for non-time-limited certificate holders did not meet with much success. Langsley (1991) noted that a
resolution passed by the American Board of Medical Specialists in 1973
calling for voluntary recertification failed to motivate large numbers of
certified specialists to become recertified. Such systems eschew the
characteristics of the 'good apples' extreme of the spectrum, but fail to
identify those who need improvement most. On the other hand, Davis *et
al.* (1990) note that formal CME programs, while producing transfer of
knowledge, often do not produce positive outcomes in improved physician performance or competence unless accompanied by reinforcement,
feedback or behaviour modification techniques.

Based on the evidence available, it is our contention that a philosophy which focuses primarily on maintenance of the competence of all practitioners, but which incorporates a system of identifying the incompetent minority who are not taking the necessary steps to improve their competence, should be adopted in any system of recertification.

A participant-centred approach to recertification has many advantages. Firstly, it values the intrinsic motivation of the practitioner to maintain competence over the external motivation provided by reward or threat. How can intrinsic motivation be generated in the practitioner? Establishing guidelines for competent practice in obstetrics and their wide dissemination were not found by Lomas *et al.* (1989) to result in rapid change in actual practice, without providing incentives or removing disincentives. Feedback on performance, while raising the awareness of the practitioner on strengths and weaknesses, will contribute towards intrinsic motivation to maintain competence for the majority, but may be unheeded by the minority who need to improve most.

A second advantage of the participant-centred approach stems from the fact that it incorporates the principles of adult learning. Adults prefer educational programmes which are flexible enough to be individualized and tailor-made to their specific needs. The diversity of any given group of doctors stems from their different practices based on individual skills and local needs. A recertification process which ignores this diversity would not assist all individuals in the group to maintain their competence in their respective practices. The societal value of recertification lies in the extent to which it evaluates each practitioner in those areas in which they actually practise, not in all the procedures encompassed by a discipline (Glassock *et al.*, 1991). A participant-centred approach encourages such individualization.

A third advantage of a participant-centred approach stems from its consonance with current approaches to education in the health professions. Placing the responsibility on the learner for identifying what is to be learnt, and for taking steps to achieve that learning is one of the cornerstones of the problem-based approach to learning. Confronting learners with a problem situation that they are likely to be faced with in practice, and letting them discover their individual gaps in knowledge or skill to deal with that situation, is surely a potent way to increase intrinsic motivation to learn and to enhance the capacity to change.

A fourth advantage of a participant-centred approach is that it encourages self-assessment and removes the threat of being judged by others. Thus it is more likely to be accepted by the majority of the practitioners.

Issues in implementation

The target group for a system of recertification should encompass all those who are involved in the practice of a discipline or specialty, not merely the incompetent few or the competent majority. In other words it will 'identify poor performance . . . improve the average and recognize the superior'. This is one of the principles adopted by the New York State Advisory Committee on Periodic Physician Recredentialing (Gellhorn, 1991). While particular attention has to be paid to special risk groups, we do not agree with the belief of the Federation of State Medical Boards of the United States that it should be required only of those practitioners who are suspected of being incompetent or who are compromised by physical or mental handicaps (see Gellhorn, 1991). McAuley (1984) has identified groups at increased risk of having unsatisfactory levels of competence. These are doctors in solo practice, who are older than 65 years, and who are neither certified by, nor members of, the relevant professional association. To these risk groups should be added those returning to practice after a period of absence and those who have undergone a career change. Also at risk are the practitioners who are so busy that they are unable to find the time to take steps to maintain their competence, and those who practise so occasionally that they may be out of touch with developments in their field. Thus, while recertification should target all practitioners in a given field, particular attention should be given to the risk groups identified above as being more likely to demonstrate inadequacy in their competence.

The responsibility for recertification has been identified above as belonging to the body that issued the certificate in the first instance. This body would vary across countries, and, to a lesser extent, across specialties within a country. The body responsible for recertification should also assume responsibility for organizing activities that assist its members to maintain competence for recertification. In many countries, bodies responsible for postgraduate medical education have concentrated on assessment at the expense of training. If recertification follows the same path the focus would be on the identification of 'bad apples' rather than on the maintenance of competence.

Any system of recertification should be subjected to intermittent evaluation to ensure that it is achieving the desired goals. Not only would evaluation enhance the credibility of the system it would also facilitate public accountability, especially if undertaken by an individual or group external to the system. Such evaluation would incorporate an analysis of the process of recertification, as well as a determination of its long-term impact on the health care provided by the practitioners.

References

Berwick, D. (1989). Continuous improvement as an ideal in health care. *New England Journal of Medicine*, **320**, 53–6.

Bowmer, M. I. (1991). 'The Canadian licensure certification muddle: a personal view'. Invited Paper, Fifth Cambridge Conference on Medical Education, Adelaide, 1991.

Davis, D. A., Norman, G. R., Painvin, A., Lindsay, E., Ragbeer, M. S. & Rath, D. (1990). Attempting to ensure physician competence. *Journal of the American Medical Association*, **263**, 2041–2.

Gellhorn, A. (1991). Periodic physician recredentialing. *Journal of the American Medical Association*, **265**, 752–5.

Glassock, R. J., Benson, J. A., Jr, Copeland, R. B., Godwin, H. A., Johanson, W. G., Point, W., Popp, R. L., Scherr, L., Stein, J. H. & Taunton, O. D. (1991). Time-limited certification and recertification: the program of the American Board of Internal Medicine. The task force on recertification. *Annals of Internal Medicine*, **114**, 59–62.

Langsley, D. G. (Editorial) (1991). Recredentialing. *Journal of the American Medical Association*, **265**, 772.

Lomas, J., Anderson, G. M., Domnick-Pierre, K., Vayda, E., Enkin, M. W. & Hannah, W. J. (1989). Do practice guidelines guide practice? The effect of a consensus statement on the practice of physicians. *New England Journal of Medicine*, **321**, 1306–11.

McAuley, R. G. (1984). Results of the Peer Assessment Program of the College of Physicians and Surgeons of Ontario. *Canadian Medical Association Journal*, **131**, 557–60.

Murchland, J. B. (1988). Quality assurance and recertification. *Australian and New Zealand Journal of Ophthalmology*, **16**, 255–7.

Silver, T. (1989). Certification and re-certification – a time and a place for action. *Journal of the Royal Society of Medicine*, **82**, 251–2.

13

Determining the content of recertification procedures

LESLEY SOUTHGATE and BRIAN JOLLY (Editors),
IAN BOWMER, DAVID NEWBLE and JOHN
NORCINI

Once recertification has become an accepted policy it follows that a process must be developed for deriving the content of the recertification which samples the appropriate domains of clinical practice and excludes items which are irrelevant or redundant (Glassock *et al.*, 1991). For example, suppose we had to recertify a particular group of specialists, there are three content-orientated questions which need to be answered.

(i) What elements of clinical practice should they be expected to perform at a very high standard?
(ii) In which tasks or features of medical practice would we not require them to be proficient?
(iii) What tasks would we expect them to perform at least as well as a competent generalist?

In order that the process of deriving this content should be useful across a wide range of clinical specialties (including the general specialties such as family practice and general internal medicine) we need to make some assumptions about the framework of clinical competence to which we are recertifying individuals.

One of the assumptions we make in this chapter is that the definition of content for recertification must be based on practitioners' competence or performance in their actual practice. It would be unreasonable to expect an expert clinician to demonstrate competence to an unrelated field for the purpose of recertification.

Another assumption we will make is that it is possible to design a strategy for deciding on the content of recertification before choosing the methods which might be used to achieve it. For example there is a tendency to equate recertification procedures with continuing medical education (CME) (Hewson, 1989; Benson, 1991; RCOG, 1991). We regard CME as only one method of achieving recertification. As the method should be chosen after the content has been defined it will, of course, be constrained by this definition. Methods are mentioned only briefly here but will be discussed more fully in the next chapter.

Finally, the purpose of recertification must be specified before the boundaries and complexity of the content can be defined adequately. Is the primary purpose concerned with identifying incompetent practitioners or is it to promote good practice? Either or both may be required at different times and will affect the recertification strategy in different ways. As the process could lead to a doctor being prevented from practising, the importance of content validity and the relevance of the assessment to actual practice is paramount. The underlying issue is the relationship between knowledge, competence and performance. Certification examinations are often dominated by tests of knowledge and have been criticized as having little relevance to actual practice (Rethans *et al.*, 1990). The evidence for the predictive validity of such examinations for subsequent performance in practice is far from convincing (Rethans *et al.*, 1991). In order to be credible, we believe that recertification procedures must ensure that the content of assessment reflects the actual content of practice and that they strive to include an assessment of actual performance in the practice setting.

In this chapter strategies for defining those aspects of clinical practice which should figure in a recertification procedure are discussed as well as organizations and individuals who should be involved in this process. Also considered briefly is how the content might shape the methods used to recertify across the spectrum of medical expertise.

The purposes of recertification

There are several potential purposes of recertification which may conflict with each other. The purpose must, however, be absolutely clear to those who are being recertified and must be determined by a wide debate within the profession and the community it serves before being implemented. Once these issues are resolved then content definition and standard setting can begin. The principal dilemma is between assessment designed to identify and eventually exclude unacceptably poor practice, and assessment designed to identify strengths and weaknesses and to promote professional development. The importance and balance given to these two aims of recertification affects the definition of content. Recertification of minimum competence and performance may emphasize a 'common core' of practice and a relatively limited range of sophisticated clinical abilities, while the promotion of good practice may require examination of the 'cutting edge' of the relevant domain. Alternatively, the content could be the same for both purposes with a different standard set for each.

A model for content determination

We see the content of recertification as being determined at four different levels (see Figure 13.1). Level 1 is a set of more or less enduring characteristics of professional medical practice which we have called the 'common core' of practice.

Levels 2 to 4 of the model express the individuality of a clinician's work, taking into account the degree of specialization evident in actual practice. The content of Level 2 is determined by the group (e.g. surgery, internal medicine) into which the practitioner was certified initially. Level 3 content is determined by an additional secondary subspecialty certification (e.g. plastic surgery; cardiology). Level 4 is the component which reflects the profile of the practitioner's day-to-day work.

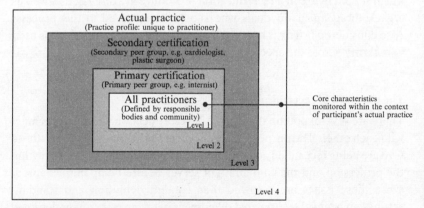

Fig. 13.1. Four-level model for the definition of the content of recertification for specialists and generalists. The model works from the common core to the outer 'shell' of actual practice.

Level 1: The common core of practice

The common core of practice is a reflection of those characteristics which distinguish an individual as a member of the medical profession. It contains the knowledge, skills and attitudes which all doctors who engage in independent practice in any branch of the profession, including the non-clinical branches, should exhibit. These include moral and ethical behaviour in the practice setting, humanistic skills, communication skills and the skills necessary to maintain competence within their chosen field. A critical approach to their own work, a willingness to engage in quality assurance activities and a commitment to independent learning are, therefore, all characteristics to be expected of any competent practitioner. The content germane to all practitioners also includes an awareness of the legal, ethical and societal issues relevant to medicine at the time of recertification. Some of the content of this common area may well be modified by society from time to time and be reflected in legislation and legal judgements.

Generally, it is accepted that recertification procedures will include the provision of evidence that the practitioner is currently in good standing with national and local licensing authorities. However, we believe it will be important to determine which aspects of the core of practice will not have been assessed by such bodies and consequently will require further attention elsewhere in the process.

It is likely that the common core of practice will be seen somewhat differently by the profession and by the state or community. The former are likely to see it as a minimum level of competence. The latter may focus on certain skills and attitudes, particularly those debated regularly in disciplinary hearings and court cases for medical negligence. Importance must be placed on the local definition of these attributes which should be culturally sensitive. Decisions about which attributes should be included in recertification must be taken within the local context. In defining the core content it will be essential to have the input of appropriate community representatives and experts in the fields of medical ethics, medical audit and communication skills.

We recommend that recertification of all clinicians should include an assessment of honesty, self-awareness in the professional context, empathy and respect for patient autonomy and confidentiality. Components of these attributes on which attention could be focused include:

Accepting feedback	Authenticity
Availability	Discretion
Flexibility	Integrity
Perseverance	Reliability
Responsibility	Sensitivity
Stamina	Tolerance
Willingness to change	

We have concluded that the common core should be assessed within the context of actual practice. For the sake of efficiency it would be appropriate to link it into Level 4 assessment. This will have implications when it comes to choosing a method of assessment.

Levels 2 and 3

Primary and secondary recertification

The way in which the content of Levels 2 and 3 is defined is fundamental to the acceptability and success of the assessment. In order that the process of doing so has the confidence of both the profession and society it must combine academic rigour with a practical understanding of local circumstances. The content should be defined by peer reference groups whose composition will vary in different countries. However, they will usually include: individuals from the primary and secondary certifying bodies; locally and nationally respected practitioners who are active currently in the clinical practice of the specialty concerned; those involved in professional development activities such as continuing medical education; members of relevant allied professions; and lay persons who are able to represent the interests of patients and society. These groups will have the task of defining the content of current practice within their domain and will use a variety of strategies including:

(i) Reviews of current work patterns, new advances and obsolete practices
(ii) An overview of the epidemiology of relevant diseases with a resulting view of need and priorities
(iii) Scrutiny of published curricula for certification in the domain and of the content of examinations used currently to assess them
(iv) Attention to changes in the context of health care in society which may change ethical guidelines and priorities and hence clinical practice

The reference group must be acknowledged as an appropriate peer group by the practitioners for whom they are defining the content of recertification. A variety of approaches to achieve credibility should be adopted (see Chapter 16). These must include wide consultation with individuals and relevant organizations. The reference groups will not necessarily determine the methods for recertification but will clearly have a direct relationship to those who do.

The generalism/specialism continuum

The practice of medicine is a continuum from generalism to specialism. The position of the individual practitioner on this continuum is determined largely by certification (primary and secondary) and by self selection, (e.g. the general practitioner who provides intrapartum care; the anaesthetist specializing in cardiac anaesthesia; the cardiologist dealing with general medicine problems). The infinite number of combinations of generalist/specialist practice found within medicine leads to problems in determining an appropriate balance for the content of recertification which we have addressed by proposing that both primary and secondary reference groups be involved. It is particularly important that the content of each component is defined by the relevant peer group and that generalists are assessed by generalists and specialists by specialists. Dialogue about content and standards should be encouraged between as well as within the reference groups but the final decisions will be taken by the group to which the dominant area of the doctor's practice belongs.

Level 4

Actual practice and the practice environment

Throughout this chapter we have emphasized the importance of relating the content of recertification to the actual practice of the doctor. This creates other problems which must be addressed, since the practice environment has a major impact on the content of the doctor's work. The local prevalence of disease, social conditions and the health care system (including the financial arrangements for care) all lead to different emphases, even within the same field of medical practice. It follows, therefore, that the content of recertification must be largely locally determined, focused on actual practice and performance-based. The definition of 'local' will be a difficult but necessary part of the work of the peer reference groups as they determine the content of recertification.

If recertification is to reflect actual practice, an element of choice of content may be necessary to allow individuals to tailor the assessment to their own practice environment. The relevant peer group must ensure that the content is sampled adequately for each individual and that choice does not lead to an overall loss of content validity. This function will be particularly important in ensuring that standards remain comparable in very different locations. The danger in this approach is that it might lead to a narrow definition of content, uneven standards and a lack of understanding and cohesion between clinicians within the same peer group.

Strategies for determining actual practice

While the broad content of recertification can be determined by the primary and secondary peer reference groups, we have concluded that the assessment should also be locally relevant and based on actual practice. Obviously it would be impossible to provide recertification options which are determined entirely by each individual's practice profile. Nevertheless, the reference groups responsible for devising the recertification procedures should provide a range of options tailored to information obtained by methods such as:

External analysis of consecutive cases
Practice log books
Referral and prescribing patterns
Direct observations
Self-identification

Combining content from different levels

The model we have advocated for determining the content of recertification may seem to be too complex to marry to a practical recertification procedure. However, we believe there are no simple or simplistic solutions if we wish the recertification procedure to be valid. The content must determine the methods to be used even if the methods currently available are inadequate. Recognizing such limitations should stimulate research aimed at the development of new ways of assessing clinical competence and clinical performance.

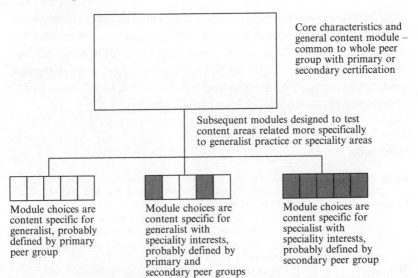

Fig. 13.2. A model to guide the assessment of primary and secondary certification content. This approach includes assessment of core characteristics, and a component related to actual practice.

It is not our brief to go into details about the methods of assessment. In broad principle, however, we envisage two arms to the recertification procedure: one based in the practice setting and one based on a more formal assessment. The latter component must be flexible enough to take into account wide variations in individual clinical practice and it can be envisaged as being developed in a modular form (see Figure 13.2). All doctors would have to complete a 'common core of practice' module. Subsequent modules would have to be designed to test the specific areas (generalist/specialist) in which the doctors practised. Thus, doctors practising in a branch of medicine defined by primary certification (e.g. family practice, surgery, internal medicine) would have to complete a general content module common to this group and doctors practising in a subspecialty would in addition have to recertify by completing modules specific to their area of practice. All practitioners would have to complete an equal number of modules but a considerable degree of choice would be allowed in order to reflect the practice profile of the individual. The content of each module would be determined by the peer reference groups referred to previously.

Achieving a valid and reliable measure of the practice-based component is one of the most difficult areas in recertification. Nevertheless, a recertification procedure without this component can never achieve long-term credibility. It would be akin to recertifying pilots without simulated or real-life checks of flying ability. Current approaches to recertification based on mandatory CME or re-examination alone cannot provide evidence of on-the-job performance, which we have identified as essential components in each level of our content model.

References

Benson, J. A. (1991). Certification and recertification: one approach to professional accountability. *Annals of Internal Medicine*, **114**, 238–42.

Glassock, R. J., Benson, J. A., Copeland, R. B., Godwin, R. B., Johanson, W. G., Point, W., Popp, R. L., Scherr, L., Stein, J. H. & Taunton, O. D. (1991). Time-limited certification and recertification: the program of the American Board of Internal Medicine. The task force on recertification. *Annals of Internal Medicine*, **114**, 59–62.

Hewson, A. D. (1989). The development of the obligatory education and certification programme of the Royal Australian College of Obstetricians and Gynaecologists: a practical response to the increasing challenges of a modern society. *Medical Teacher*, **11**, 27–37.

RCOG (Royal College of Obstetricians and Gynaecologists) (1991). *Report of the Working Party on Continuing Medical Education*. London: Royal College of Obstetricians and Gynaecologists.

Rethans, J. J., Sturmans, F., Drop, R., van der Vleuten, C. & Hobus, P. (1991). Does competence of general practitioners predict performance? Comparison between examination setting and actual practice. *British Medical Journal*, **303**, 1377–80.

Rethans, J., van Leeuwen, Y., Drop, R., Sturmans, F. & van der Vleuten, C. (1990). Competence and performance: two different constructs in the assessment of the quality of medical care. *Family Practice*, **7**, 168–74.

14

Methods of assessment in recertification

RICHARD HAYS (Editor), WAYNE DAVIS, BETH
DAWSON-SAUNDERS, ELIZABETH FARMER,
JOHN FOULKES, GARETH HOLSGROVE,
DONALD LANGSLEY, COLIN McRAE, PETER
PROCOPIS and ARTHUR ROTHMAN

The expectation that individual medical practitioners should demonstrate a continuing level of competence throughout their careers poses a major opportunity as well as a challenge to policy-makers and medical education researchers. New methods of assessment need to be developed to measure performance of a group of highly trained professionals who have progressed beyond supervision in training institutions and the tests of knowledge appropriate to certification of competence. The profession's policy-makers must work together with test developers to create methods which satisfy validity, reliability and efficiency requirements, and are acceptable to members of the profession.

Selection of methods will depend on many contextual factors related to the discipline and how it is practised, the purpose of the assessment and how it is to be implemented. These issues have been discussed in detail in earlier chapters. Because each discipline may have to approach recertification methods differently, this chapter outlines a generic process for determining the most appropriate methods of assessment. Examples of how to apply this process to three different disciplines, rural general/family practitioners, specialist surgeons in private practice and paediatricians in an academic institution, will be provided.

Principles for selection of assessment methods

Although several methods of assessment are currently available, their application to recertification assessment is not clear and the temptation to

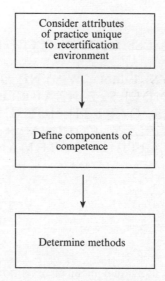

Fig. 14.1. Process for selection of assessment methods appropriate for recertification.

simply select one of those methods should be resisted. The preferred approach is: to consider attributes of professional practice unique to the recertification environment; to use the actual practice of individual members of the discipline to define components of competence (the content) to be assessed; and then to select or to develop appropriate methods. This process is represented in Figure 14.1.

The recertification environment

Recertification assessment and certification assessment have several contextual differences. Candidates for recertification are experienced clinicians who tend to work in specific content disciplines in autonomous or semi-autonomous situations. They are dispersed geographically, creating logistic difficulties in organization of the assessment. Some may not be convinced of the need for recertification assessment. Successful recertification programmes require professional organizations to ensure that newly certified clinicians are aware that they have not been awarded career-long credentials. Policy-makers will need to be clear about the purpose of the assessment, whether to detect incompetence in some or to improve performance in all practitioners, as each may require different approaches in both methods and standards, and may have different social and legal consequences. These broad policy considerations have been discussed in more detail in Chapter 12.

While specific recommendations regarding appropriate methods are not possible without consideration of the context in which recertification occurs, some general guidelines can be formulated. This paper assumes that policy-makers who need to adopt methods for recertification will have considered these issues fully before proceeding to selection of assessment methods.

Defining components of competence for recertification

One approach in determining components of competence is to identify a large number of clinical tasks within the range of competence of the particular practice discipline, and then to measure performance on a sample of those tasks (see also Chapter 6). The broader the discipline (e.g. general/family practice) the more difficult this becomes. Although all clinicians will require a common core of knowledge, skills and general attributes, assessing competence to continue practising in each discipline may be directed more appropriately at those components of competence unique to each discipline (see also Chapter 13). As an example, recertification for neurologists and surgeons should require assessment of different knowledge and skill content.

Three strategies for determining the components of competence may be employed, each within the specific context of the discipline and purpose of the recertification process. The first strategy uses existing data related to practitioner behaviour. Table 14.1 lists data which may already be available from employers, funding authorities, government, and professional groups. For example, data on the range of services provided, drugs prescribed, referrals made to other disciplines and costs incurred may be available. An inherent problem is that such data are collected for other purposes, and may be in a form not immediately applicable to assessment of professional competence.

The second strategy uses empirical methods to record what practitioners actually do. This may be more appropriate where there is greater variation in what doctors do, as in general/family practice. Descriptive research, such as arranging for a sample of practitioners to record their activities in logbooks or permitting direct observation of their activities,

Table 14.1. *Data which may be currently collected and available to assist in defining components of competence*

Mortality data
Morbidity data
Referral patterns
Prescribing profiles
Participation in CME (as either learner or teacher)
Service delivery patterns
Clinical investigations profiles
Complaints by peers or patients to professional boards
Patient surveys
Critical incident surveys
Performance in management of particular diseases, e.g. diabetes
Audit of procedures performed
Involvement in local hospitals
Research grants awarded and papers published

CME is continuing medical education.

can assist in determining competencies required. Similarly, critical incident studies can identify key competencies which have an impact on the outcome of health care (Flanagan, 1954; Hubbard *et al.*, 1965).

The third strategy uses rational methods to determine competencies. For example, task analyses or Delphi methods may be employed to generate a list of activities in which the particular practitioner should demonstrate competence (Neufeld & Norman, 1985). This approach can be from the perspective of the particular discipline concerned, or can incorporate views of other groups, such as other health professionals and health care consumers.

These three strategies may produce different perspectives on the components of competence required for a particular discipline. Combining two or all three strategies may be appropriate therefore in certain circumstances to generate the desired broad understanding of competence. The preceding chapter has dealt with the issue of determining the content to be assessed in more detail and in a somewhat different manner. Irrespective of the strategy adopted to define the content of the recertification procedure, assessment methods must be sought which match the content. While this may appear self-evident, it is not uncommon for the reverse to be the case with the assessment method determining the content.

Table 14.2. *Methods of assessment in recertification in assumed
ascending order of validity*

Multiple-choice questions
Written tests (essays, short answers)
Oral exams (vivas)
Simulated patient cases
Peer/patient review
Practice audit
Direct observation

Determining methods

In determining methods appropriate to the tasks requiring assessment,
policy-makers should consider the full range of methods currently available as well as seek new approaches (Neufeld & Norman, 1985; Wakeford, 1985). Certain methods assess different components of competence
better than others; for example procedural skills and cognitive skills
require quite different approaches to assessment. The ideal method of
assessing clinical performance is one which is easy to administer,
measures the appropriate components of competence (is valid), produces
reproducible results (is reliable), and is efficient in terms of resources.

Table 14.2 lists available assessment methods. It may be assumed that
this reflects ascending order of validity at the recertification level (see also
Chapter 8). Most methods currently in use in undergraduate and certification examinations rate poorly as appropriate methods for the purposes
of recertification.

The focus of assessment in medical education is currently moving.
Assessment of competence in terms of knowledge alone is no longer
regarded as appropriate. How professionals apply their knowledge is
recognized as the key indicator of competence (Norman *et al.*, 1990). The
nearer assessment approaches measurement of performance, the more
valid will be that assessment, particularly where the subjects of assessment are experienced practitioners (Miller, 1990). 'Experts' appear to
behave differently from 'novices' by making intuitive leaps in diagnosis
based on the experience of having seen conditions before (Schmidt *et al.*,
1990). New methods may have to be developed to assess what experienced practitioners actually do, rather than what they can do in written or

simulated situations, and the format of the assessment should be derived from actual practice.

Application of the process to three example disciplines

A knowledge of what is actually done by practitioners in a particular discipline may make it possible to develop new, or to adapt old, methods of assessment for the recertification context. This is illustrated by discussing recertification in three disciplines. In preparing these examples there is an underlying assumption that the purpose of the assessment is primarily educational and developmental rather than punitive, aiming to improve quality of care provided by all practitioners. The focus of the assessment in each example is recertification to continue practising in the relevant discipline. Other contextual variables are outlined for each case. Only methods considered to have the potential to be valid in recertification are discussed.

The general family practitioner

As the scope of general/family practice is so broad, a combination of existing data, empirical and rational approaches to defining competence may be necessary to ensure that all aspects of practice and their impact on the health care of the community are considered. Choice of methods will be determined initially by acceptability, feasibility, cost, and whether the implementation is voluntary or mandatory. As practices will vary according to the scope and the availability of support services, the context of the practitioner's own practice will determine the measures needed to demonstrate competence. Clearly, the assessment should be practice-based and, where possible, on-site. Distance itself may not be an issue in determining assessment methods; at a cost, distance barriers can be overcome by use of modern communications technology and by on-site visits.

Discussed below in ascending order of validity are possible methods appropriate for assessing competence in the family practice situation.

Records of achievement

Records of achievement constitute a portfolio of actual practice data covering desired competencies. This could include self audit of clinical cases managed (both procedural and non-procedural), hospital privileges gained, participation in continuing medical education (CME) activities, and involvement in research. Although mere participation in CME or research does not necessarily mean change in practice behaviour, an assessment of the impact of the activity on an individual's practice may provide useful information (Beaudry, 1989).

Computerized evaluation methods

Using a personal computer and a modem, isolated practitioners could access knowledge-based tests and computerized simulations which could be used for either educational or recertification purposes. Such a scheme is already in operation in Australia (Marshall, 1989).

External audit

Practice audit is now common in general practice in the United Kingdom, where most practices have installed a sophisticated computer suited to this task (Baker, 1991). Trained visiting auditors could conduct in-depth analyses of how the practice and the individual practitioner compare with agreed standards on such measures as chart audits of immunization rates, cervical screening rates, prescribing, or referrals to other health services. The effectiveness of chart audits may be limited by the quality of medical records. Review of letters of admission to hospital from general practitioners has met with some success (Hughes, 1991).

Assessment by standardized patients

Consenting clinicians could be advised that they would be consulted during a specified time period by standardized patients who would not identify themselves. Such standardized patients could assess communication skills or management of specific tracer conditions. Successful trials of such schemes have been reported (Rethans *et al.*, 1991).

Direct observation by trained assessors

Trained observers could visit and observe the consultations of the general practitioner, as already happens in the vocational training programme in Australia (Hays, 1990). Education/assessment visits by colleagues in similar circumstances could be arranged (Ward, 1989; Grol, 1990). A variation on direct observation, tried without success in certification assessment and to be used in trials in recertification assessment, is assessment of videotaped genuine consultations from an individual's practice (Hays *et al.*, 1990). A key issue yet to be determined is the duration of observation and the number and range of cases that need to be observed to form a reliable judgement of performance. In the rural context, specialists sometimes visit isolated practices to provide a mixture of clinical service and on-site education for the doctors. The role of these visits could be expanded to include formal reports of interactions with the practitioner, provided that the visiting specialists were trained to perform this task. For example, a visiting obstetrician/gynaecologist may observe a delivery or gynaecological procedure undertaken by the practitioner and make an assessment.

The surgeon in private practice

Development of methods for recertification of the surgeon in private practice must, as in all groups, take into account the specific context in which metropolitan surgeons practise. Surgeons function in a specialty environment of some specificity and rely on other disciplines for assist-ance in the management of the breadth of medicine and surgery. Therefore it may be easier to determine their activities, and it may be possible to develop recertification methods that are more practice specific than for broader specialties. Their practice is, however, less supervised than that of hospital-based colleagues. Private practice surgeons will be consulted in their own offices, may interact with a number of hospitals for inpatient surgical activity, and may even own a day surgical facility. To this extent, private practice surgeons and private general practitioners have similar practice styles.

At present there is no clear definition of surgical competence, although some adverse outcome measurements have been used to attempt to identify inadequate performance. Development of recertification methods will be difficult until more definition of what constitutes com-petence becomes available.

Areas that may be considered for the assessment of competence of private practice surgeons include knowledge, diagnostic, procedural and communication skills. All are to some extent specialty and subspecialty specific. Little attempt has been made to assess communication skills of surgeons even though inadequacies in these skills are a major source of patient complaints. Although there are existing data on the incidence of such complaints, only a small number of surgeons who are performing inadequately are identified, and currently this is not sufficient to be a method of general elevation of performance.

Some methods of assessment that could be used, in ascending order of validity, are discussed below.

Involvement in continuing medical education (CME)

Recording participation in continuing medical education is a relatively simple and feasible method which is likely to be acceptable to surgeons. A wide variety of activities are available and appropriate – scientific meetings, workshops, journal clubs, private journal reading, self-assessment programmes, etc. Participation in CME is often required for accreditation for clinical privileges in surgical facilities. Ensuring adequate involvement in CME by metropolitan surgeons could be a useful method of ensuring maintenance of knowledge and its current application in surgery, although defining and assessing adequacy of involvement in CME may be difficult (Beaudry, 1989).

Patient surveys

Patient satisfaction is an important aspect of surgical outcome, although there is little evidence that measuring patient satisfaction improves health care (Vuori, 1991). There may be some potential to develop measures of satisfaction further, in particular for communication skills and quality of outcome of surgical procedures, although care must be taken with interpretation of data as relationships between patient and surgeon may influence the assessment.

Peer review

Review of competency by peers may be seen as one of the least threatening methods, although review committees must ensure that judgements are based on valid and reliable information. Credentialing committees composed of surgical peers could be established by every hospital to review performance of individual surgeons regularly. Such committees could use audit data, content and frequency of complaints, and health status in assessing continuing competence.

Surgical audit

Audit requires the accurate collection of data on aspects of surgical practice that are related to the quality of patient care, regular review by peers of such data and a mechanism for change when necessary. Considerable resources are required for the introduction of audit into surgical departments, as is a substantial degree of commitment for its continued use. Unfortunately, many of the areas chosen for audit have not been validated relative to the quality of patient care and more development is needed here. Despite these concerns, involvement in surgical audit may offer one of the best prospects of improving the overall performance of surgeons.

Practice profiles and activity analyses

Relative incidences of specific procedures may be of use in assessing competence. Although this needs to be interpreted in the context of the individual surgeon's practice, large variations between practice profiles of individuals compared with peers may enable unacceptable performance to be identified.

Direct observation

Surgeons are observed routinely by anaesthetists, assistants and nursing staff, and, in larger institutions, may also be observed by peers and trainee surgeons. Information from these sources could be assessed by peer review committees. Methods will need to be devised to standardize and collect these data. Appropriate instruments will have to be constructed. There are significant hurdles to overcome, although the potential is substantial.

The paediatrician in a teaching hospital

Paediatricians in teaching hospitals work in an environment which differs from those of the previous two examples. They practise within large institutions with strong links to universities. Clinical practice, teaching and research are expected to be complementary roles, and activities are expected to reflect the leading edge of practice in paediatrics. Academic staff have responsibility for teaching both undergraduate and graduate students, and are expected to act as a resource for other paediatricians as well as generalists working in other environments.

Differences between paediatric teaching hospitals and their adult counterparts must be recognized. Although the range of services and subspecialties offered equates with the larger adult hospitals, paediatric hospitals are usually smaller in size, have a significantly shorter average length of stay and a large outpatient service component. Therefore, methods of assessment may need to rely more on outpatient (ambulatory) care services than in other specialist disciplines.

In formulating methods of assessment for recertification, a combination of existing data sources and recording activities of clinicians may be of assistance. Most paediatric teaching hospitals have active quality assurance programmes in place (e.g. Australian Council for Hospital Standards Accreditation Guide, 1991) which could be modified easily to define components of competence through task analysis. Methods of assessment could be adapted from the inevitable scrutiny that clinical staff are under within an academic institution.

Possible methods appropriate for assessing competence in ascending order of assumed validity are discussed below.

Clinical knowledge

Clinical knowledge of academic clinicians could be assessed by methods available to non-academic paediatricians. For example, clinical knowledge could be self-assessed by structured multiple-choice questions with appropriate feedback, such as that undertaken for recertification by the American Board of Pediatrics (Brownlee, 1987). Content will vary according to the subspeciality being assessed. Self-assessment programmes, because of the resources required, would be carried out best on a national basis by the appropriate specialty organization.

Audit of clinical activities

Formal audit of clinical cases seen or procedures performed may be adapted to indicate components of competence required in individual subspecialities. Each subspeciality will have different components of competence. Existing databases may, with minimal alteration, produce acceptable performance indicators. For example, the performance of general paediatricians in the management of specific childhood illnesses, such as asthma, could be monitored using objective criteria such as mode of treatment, patient understanding, and assessment of long- and short-term outcome (Bucknall *et al.*, 1988).

Stimulated chart recall

Quality of care criteria could also be formulated and assessed by stimulated chart recall (Munger & Reinhart, 1987). The validity of such performance indicators may be open to question, since there are numerous variables in addition to the individual academic clinician in charge of management (e.g. severity of symptoms, junior staff involvement, etc.). However, aggregated data from a large number of cases may produce valuable information. Studies using such criteria have shown lower morbidity in patients treated by specialist units as compared to non-specialist units in the same hospital (Bucknall *et al.*, 1988). Not all existing data will be of use. Crude mortality and morbidity data are unlikely to be useful except for the confirmation of the grossly incompetent practitioner.

Audit of teaching and research

Teaching and research activities may also be assessed, since they are essential to the role of the clinician in the academic environment. Existing methods of assessing performance in research (number and value of grants, number and status of publications) and teaching (student and peer assessments) could be employed (Hilliard, 1990).

Peer review

Although peer review ratings provide a broad overview of competence only, some validity of assessment has been shown (Ramsay *et al.*, 1989). Clinicians in academic institutions are in an environment where performance is under scrutiny from peers, postgraduate and undergraduate students. Regular attendance and active participation in hospital clinical meetings, journal club and special society meetings is expected, with individual staff members required to present clinical cases and to discuss recent developments in the research literature. All cases resulting in the death of patients are reviewed by mortality review committees where qualitative information behind crude mortality statistics is discussed. It may be possible to devise assessment methods based on participation in these meetings and observation by peers. For example, a global rating

Table 14.3. *Some research issues concerning recertification*

Validity as predictors of continuing competence of peer ratings, multiple-choice questions, standardized patients and self-evaluation
Does feedback affect performance in the clinical situation?
The effect on performance of trained itinerant clinician-assessors in isolated/rural practice
Defining discipline-related practice content
Self-assessed vs. actual needs for continuing education
Defining real patient outcomes
Application of the meta-analytic approach to recertification

scale commenting on willingness to discuss errors, awareness of the current literature and ability to accept constructive feedback could be devised for completion by peers.

Conclusion

Assessment for recertification purposes represents a new phase in medical education research and development. Determining appropriate methods of assessment requires: consideration of the different context in which experienced medical practitioners work; the definition of relevant components of competence; and the findings of methods to match both context and content. No single method can provide a comprehensive measure of competence. Just as certification assessment requires a battery of tests, recertification assessment needs an approach which combines different methods for different aspects of practice.

Implementation of recertification cannot wait until all remaining questions have been answered. Policy-makers must implement recertification programmes based on information currently available and must make a commitment to future research and development. Some high priority research issues are listed in Table 14.3. In particular, methods which measure actual performance of practitioners against real health-care outcomes are required.

References

Australian Council for Hospital Standards Accreditation Guide (1991). *Standards for Australian Health Care Facilities*, 10th edn. Sydney: ACHS.
Baker, R. (1991). Audit and standards in new general practice. *British Medical Journal*, **303**, 32–4.

Beaudry, J. S. (1989). The effectiveness of continuing medical education: a quantitative analysis. *The Journal of Continuing Education*, **9**, 285–307.

Brownlee, R. C. (1987). Recertification examinations linked to CME. In *Recertification of Medical Specialists*, ed. J. S. Lloyd & D. G. Langsley, pp. 43–8. Evanston: American Board of Medical Specialties.

Bucknall, C. A., Robertson, C., Moran, F. & Stevenson, R. D. (1988). Differences in hospital asthma management. *Lancet*, **i**, 748–50.

Flanagan, J. C. (1954). The critical incident technique. *Psychological Bulletin*, **51**, 327–58.

Grol, R. (1990). Peer review in primary care. *Quality Assurance in Health Care*, **2**, 119–26.

Hays, R. B. (1990). A training program for rural general practice. *Medical Journal of Australia*, **153**, 546–8.

Hays, R. B., Jones, B. F., Adkins, P. B. & McKain, P. J. (1990). Analysis of videotaped consultations to certify competence. *Medical Journal of Australia*, **152**, 609–11.

Hilliard, R. I. (1990). The good and effective teacher as perceived by paediatric residents and faculty. *American Journal of Diseases in Childhood*, **144**, 1106–10.

Hubbard, J. P., Levit, E. J., Schumacher, C. F. & Schnabel, T. G. (1965). An objective evaluation of clinical competence. *New England Journal of Medicine*, **272**, 1321–8.

Hughes, C. (1991). Quality assurance in the Swan District Hospital. *Australian Clinical Review*, **11**, 103–5.

Marshall, J. R. (1989). CHECKUP. Computerised home evaluation of clinical knowledge understanding and problem-solving. *Teaching and Learning in Medicine*, **1**, 38–41.

Miller, G. E. (1990). The assessment of clinical skills/competence/performance. *Academic Medicine*, **65** (supplement), 63–7.

Munger, B. S. & Reinhart, M. A. (1987). Field trial of multiple recertification methods. In *Recertification of Medical Specialists*, ed. J. S. Lloyd & D. G. Langsley, pp. 71–8. Evanston: American Board of Medical Specialties.

Neufeld, V. R. & Norman, G. R. (Eds.) (1985). *Assessing Clinical Competence*. New York: Springer.

Norman, G., Allery, L., Berkson, L., *et al.* (1990) 'The psychology of clinical reasoning: implications for assessment'. Paper presented at the Fourth Cambridge Conference. Cambridge University School of Clinical Medicine.

Ramsay, P. G., Carline, J. D., Inui, T. S., Larson, E. B., LoGerfo, J. P. & Wenrich, M. D. (1989). Predictive validity of certification by the American Board of Internal Medicine. *Annals of Internal Medicine*, **110**, 719–26.

Rethans, J. J., van der Vleuten, C., Drop, R. & Sturmans, F. (1991). Assessment of performance of general practitioners by the use of standardized (simulated) patients. *British Journal of General Practice*, **41**, 97–9.

Schmidt, H. G., Norman, G. R. & Boshuizen, H. P. A. (1990). A cognitive perspective on medical expertise: theory and implications. *Academic Medicine*, **65**, 611–21.

Vuori, H. (1991). Patient satisfaction – does it matter? *Quality Assurance in Health Care*, **3**, 183–9.

Wakeford, R. (Ed.) (1985). *Directions in Clinical Assessment*. Cambridge: Cambridge School of Clinical Medicine.

Ward, J. (1989). Interpractice visits by colleagues. A future option for Quality Assurance? *Australian Family Physician*, **18**, 1056–60.

15

Standard setting for recertification

DALE DAUPHINEE (Editor), SUSAN CASE,
WESLEY FABB, PAULINE McAVOY,
NICHOLAS SAUNDERS and RICHARD
WAKEFORD

The notion of recertification for doctors in active medical practice is gaining wide acceptance (see Chapters 4 and 5). While the concept of having to establish one's credentials on a regular basis is most attractive to the casual observer, the operational consequences of implementing such a system are major tasks. More importantly, certain aspects of assessing for recertification present challenges which are not issues in the most traditional settings for certification. To start, one has to contend with the problem of variable content of the examination if it is to be practice-specific. However, perhaps most challenging is the absence of a cohort effect when establishing standards. Both problems are a direct result of the highly individualistic nature of the patient and problem profiles in doctor's practices: varied populations, varied environmental factors, varied social conditions, varied health problems, to name a few of the parameters. Thus, if the content of the recertification is to reflect what the doctor does, a flexible process will be needed. Unlike those in postgraduate clinical training programmes or medical students in a graduating class who have gone through a prescribed curriculum and a similar set of clinical experiences, candidates for recertification have lost the traditional class or cohort effect of clinical training so that defining a reference group or criteria for standard setting may present a significant challenge to the recertifying agency.

This is not to suggest that the task is impossible. Rather, one must anticipate the challenge and be prepared to make choices as how to deal with standard setting in these conditions. Our purpose in this chapter is not to write a cookery book but rather to provide a map: the reader will decide the destinations (goals) and which roads (methods) to take.

At the outset, the authors of the assessment process must determine the purpose of recertification. Specifically the evaluation should identify:

(i) Those whose educational or professional practice/performance is acceptable and therefore who can be recertified

(ii) Those whose educational or professional practice/performance is either dangerous or below standard but not necessarily dangerous, or whose recertification should be deferred

(iii) In all instances, the areas in which practitioners need remediation

As a final introductory comment, let us recall that all forms of assessment constitute two principal steps: gathering data which involves measurement, and a judgement or conclusion about the meaning of that data. There is a tendency to forget that, even in multiple-choice examinations, for which accurate raw scores can be generated, a decision is necessary about the pass/fail point. The second step can be made using one of several methods, but it always involves making a judgement and therefore is subjective. This discussion focuses on the second step: how to make a judgement about the pass/fail standard for a recertification process.

Before dealing with methods, a review of definitions and key concepts is necessary.

Definitions, key concepts and approaches

In thinking about establishing a pass/fail standard for recertification, two types of assessment methods can be considered: a traditional examination approach (e.g. multiple-choice type test or standardized oral exam) or a practice-based approach (e.g. audit of practice looking at charts, outcome measures, surveying patients).

As background, a brief introduction to the approaches and terms used in standard setting is essential (see also Chapters 6 and 9). While it is estimated that there are dozens of methods to set standards (Berk, 1986), there are two basic types of standards: relative and absolute. In relative standards, whether examinees pass or fail depends on their performance relative to others who are taking the examination (e.g. those who fail are either the bottom 20% of candidates or those who score more than 15% below the mean). Absolute standards are established independently of the performance of the group that is taking an examination, (e.g. 70% correct or above is a pass). A third type, compromise methods, involves a combination of absolute and relative standards (for more detail see Berk, 1986).

What process should be used to establish the pass/fail point?

As noted, the process of establishing a pass/fail standard involves the use of both data and judgement. In the context of recertification, we favour the idea of some form of a sequential testing involving the initial use of a screening test to identify clearly deficient individuals. Those who pass the first hurdle would progress to subsequent and more finely tuned assessments. The standard should take into account the consequences of failing someone who should have passed and conversely of passing someone who should have failed.

It is being suggested that the standard be established by a content-based approach (absolute or criterion-referenced) tempered as necessary by relative standard or norm-referenced considerations (i.e. it may or may not be appropriate to pass everyone; it seems clearly inappropriate to fail a very large proportion of the examinees). A compromise method between the content-based and norm-referenced approaches, such as proposed by Hofstee (1983), may be more appropriate.

Who should be in the reference group?

If using either relative or compromise methods, to evaluate the fairness of a pass/fail standard some reference group should be identified. In specialty board certification, this group is often defined as consisting of individuals who have completed an approved training progamme and who are taking the examination for the first time. For recertification, the reference group might be defined to include individuals who are applying for recertification for the first time and who were certified originally within the past 10 or 15 years, and who have some particular practice profile. The primary issue is that the reference group must include a population with known characteristics whose performance can be used to judge whether or not the established pass/fail standard is appropriate.

Should standard setting be based on individual components or on global assessment?

If the assessment involves multiple components (particularly in the practice-based approach), scoring based on the sum of the components may not reflect the overall adequacy of the performance by an individual (see Chapter 10). For example, the component score may be adequate but may hide major deficits in specific areas which are cancelled by very high scores in other aspects.

While there is some comfort in appearing precise, there is some danger in overquantification or fragmenting the scoring into many small components not reflective of reality and possibly lacking validity. Thus, when making a decision on a standard, one must decide if the standard is to be set based on a score from many individual components or a global score or both. There is some evidence derived from a study of essay-marking techniques that global assessments may be more reliable than summing component ratings (Norcini *et al.*, 1990). It is suggested that, somehow, a global judgement should be included in assessing the quality of performance.

Challenges in recertification

The ways in which standard setting might need to be different for recertification as compared to certification should be considered. On the other hand, methods of standard setting will be modified according to the assessment processes used in recertification, just as in certification.

Standard setting as a derivative of the recertification process

There are two broad approaches to recertification:

 (i) The use of assessment procedures which test clinical competence
(ii) The assessment of the level and quality of participation in maintenance of competence programmes, which are, first and foremost, educational

With both approaches, decisions will be pass/fail, and in practice 'fail' will equate with 'defer', since there is general agreement that those not reaching the standard should be given further time to reach it. Hence, the notion of starting the recertification process in advance of the deadline is advised (e.g. start in the seventh year of a 10-year certification cycle).

Although recertification processes need to examine the 'big picture' rather than the fine detail, the process should be capable of providing specific and timely feedback which can be used for remedial learning.

Standard setting for common assessment procedures

A variety of standard-setting procedures are available (see Table 15.1). These have been discussed in detail in Chapters 9 and 10. For example

Table 15.1. *Approaches to standard setting*

Methods	Example/reference
Traditional 'gut' methods (not recommended)	Percentage correct – e.g. 50% Fail certain number Automatic failure for major gap(s) in knowledge/skills
Group performance-based standards Equating tests	Use questions or examination given to another stable group: equate standard (Holmes, 1986)
Norm referenced	Specific percentile on reference group is pass/fail mark (Schumacher, 1978)
Rating cases and global judgement	Oral examination with panel (McLean *et al.*, 1988)
Content-based standards (absolute) Nedelsky	Judge which response on each item the minimally competent could dismiss as incorrect (Nedelsky, 1954)
Ebel	Rate each item on two dimensions; construct table for test; judge each cell re percentage correct (Ebel, 1979)
Angoff	Judge each test item: estimate probability that minimum competent person would answer it correctly (Angoff, 1971)
Compromise method Hofstee	Judges specify four values for written test and standard is intercept between model and real curve (see Figure 15.1) (Hofstee, 1983)

(see Table 15.1), they include absolute content-based standards (like the Nedelsky, Ebel or Angoff methods) or compromise methods (like the Hofstee method, see Figure 15.1).

Multiple-choice tests (MCQ)

If enough questions on a recertification MCQ examination are common with an existing certification MCQ examination, these can be used for 'equating' the standards for recertification with those for certification (see

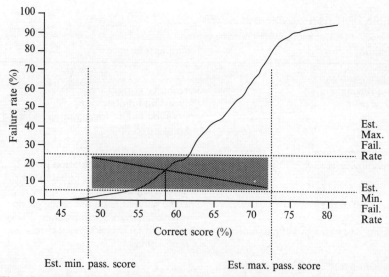

Fig. 15.1. Hofstee compromise method of standard setting. This example has identified 58% as the minimum passing score. To obtain this score, judges review the examination and estimate four values: lowest and highest acceptable passing scores (est. min. pass. score and est. max. pass. score); lowest and highest acceptable failure rates (est. min. fail. rate and est. max. fail. rate). The examinee performance curve is plotted showing possible failure rates as a function of actual scores. Two points (the intersection between est. min. pass. score and est. max. fail. rate and that of est. max. pass. score and est. min. fail. rate) are plotted and joined as demonstrated by the diagonal line in the figure. The standard is set at the point of intersection with the curve.

Table 15.1). The pass/fail line could be set higher or lower than for certification, but would be linked to it.

Oral and clinical tests

Such tests seem likely to be chosen for recertification, if on no other grounds than their face validity. There seems to be little possibility of equating such recertification tests with their certification counterparts. Moreover, it may be that recertification orals and clinicals will seek different data.

Therefore, standards could be set using the above-mentioned methods but, if global judgements are preferred rather than summing component ratings, standards and pass/fail decisions may best be established by the collective judgement of experts. They may decide on the level of performance required for recertification and the type of behaviour which represent dangerous practice, which in itself may be sufficient to defer recertification, even if the individual has reached the required standard otherwise. In these situations standard setting is being incorporated into scoring or assessment.

Social and political issues in recertification

Who should determine the pass/fail standard?

The standard for recertification should be established by the same group which identifies the actual pass/fail point for the examination. This group can appropriately obtain information from a variety of sources such as peers, other members of the health-care team and patients. The group should use this information in making a judgement about an appropriate pass/fail standard.

Implications of a failing decision

The process should allow for a period of remediation rather than immediate removal of someone's certification. For example, the process could allow individuals several attempts before their certification expires. If the original certification was a 10-year period of time, attempts to obtain recertification could be permitted after seven years.

Feedback to candidates

It seems important to provide more than just a pass/fail decision or a single score. Feedback, at least for failers, should be detailed enough to be useful for remediation. However, it is highly likely that some passing candidates will also want feedback. Hence, feedback on strengths and weaknesses may be desirable, if feasible, for all takers.

How much data should be collected prior to making a pass/fail decision?

Flexibility could be built into the system to allow pass/fail decisions to be made on variable numbers of cases or items. It is possible that some examinees will be so clearly substandard that a pass/fail judgement can be made with fewer questions/cases. For those who are closer to the pass/fail point, an extended or sequential procedure may be needed.

Table 15.2. *Typical examination methods and possible approaches to standard setting*

Examination method	Score	Methods of standard setting
MCQ (certifying)	Yes	Norm referenced Angoff Compromise method Test equating
MCQ (recertification)	Yes (with focus on practice content)	As for MCQ (certifying)
Standardized case oral (written case history with structure to examination)	Pass/fail per case (avoid checklists; need criteria/case)	Implicit with panel (with judges or peers) Percentage pass (sum-up) Angoff with Hofstee
OSCE format (including standardized patient)	Checklist score with implicit judgements, re pass/fail	Angoff Collective judgements

Examples of recertification procedures

At this juncture, it may be of value to illustrate the approach to standard setting with two examples. The first is an approach taken by a surgical specialty board and the second is the proposed scheme being considered by a national primary care organization. Both examples can be viewed as cases for discussion in which the reader can consider other approaches which could be used if these scenarios were applied to their local circumstances (see Table 15.2).

Example A: Recertification by the American Board of Orthopaedic Surgery (ABOS)

To illustrate the recertification process within a specialty board, the American Board of Orthopaedic Surgery (ABOS) has been selected as an example. In 1986, the ABOS began granting time-limited certification; all certificates granted by the ABOS are now valid for 10 years. It should be stressed that recertification, as well as certification, is a voluntary activity.

In 1990, the President of the ABOS outlined his perspective on recertification. He emphasized that the evaluation should measure whether or not an orthopaedist has kept pace with advances in the field; that anyone who has kept pace should pass (i.e. the standard should not be norm-referenced); and that the process should require enough effort to ensure that its value is recognized. While recertification has been offered by the ABOS for at least 10 years, it is expected that the numbers of candidates will increase significantly as the first cohort of examinees face the need to renew their certification.

In order to be recertified by the ABOS, a candidate must have been certified by the ABOS previously and must have a valid medical license. In addition, the candidate must: complete an application form; satisfy the continuing education requirements; and complete one of the evaluation options successfully. In reviewing the application form, the Credentials Committee of the ABOS reviews information and recommendations submitted by the candidate and may visit the practice of a candidate if that is deemed necessary. Since 1993, there are three evaluation options: a practice-based oral examination; a proctored multiple-choice test focusing on recent developments in orthopaedic surgery; and a practice audit. A candidate may elect to take any of the three evaluation options. Upon failure of any one assessment the candidate may continue to take any of the three options over the course of four years following a single application. A fourth evaluation option planned for the future is a practice-tailored multiple-choice examination, possibly computer administered.

The practice-based oral examination

The practice-based oral examination requires that candidates submit a list of operative procedures (in-hospital, ambulatory and office) performed over a six-month period. This list is organized according to 10 surgical categories and the candidate must select one case from each category for the examination. Candidates must bring to the examination all X-rays, admission and discharge notes, and office notes for each of the 10 cases, plus copies of the complete case list. They will be seen by several examiners, who may quiz the candidate on any of the 10 cases or any case included on the case list. The examiners meet to determine the overall pass/fail decision. If they are unable to arrive at a decision, the candidate will be examined by a new panel of examiners.

The general multiple-choice examination

This examination consists of 150 multiple-choice questions. The content focuses on recent developments in orthopaedic surgery that all certified orthopaedists are expected to know, regardless of their practice profile or subspecialty. Most of the items will be phrased within the context of a patient scenario, and will include relevant patient history, physical examination, and laboratory results; most will also be accompanied by relevant X-rays or other visual material. Rather than being asked to recall isolated facts, examinees will be asked to indicate the most likely diagnosis or the most appropriate next step in management.

The practice audit

The practice audit examination is a personal examination conducted by two examiners over a two-day period at the candidate's office. Candidates must submit a 12-month case list to the ABOS which selects cases for detailed review. The ABOS has noted that failure in the practice audit may require reporting the results to the state and national licensing and quality control authorities.

The standards

The standards for the practice-based oral examination and the practice audit are determined implicitly by the examiners. Examiners will be expected to use an absolute standard, determining whether or not the candidate has demonstrated sufficient knowledge and skills to be recertified. There will be no failing or passing quota. Standard-setting procedures for the general multiple-choice examination have not been determined. It is likely, however, that several pieces of information will be considered in determining a pass/fail point.

Example B: Recertification by a national college of general practitioners

A national college of general practitioners is considering a recertification process. They have not established their final procedure but are proposing an approach utilizing four components, discussed below.

Chart audit

This component will consist of 80 office cases selected randomly from the practice of the doctor under review. Of this sample, 40 patients will be surveyed. From these, 20 consenting patients will have their charts reviewed by the visiting site team. The team will assess the charts for the quality of records and management. In addition, from the original 80 charts selected at random, an audit of practice targets will be done. For example, immunization rates could be assessed against standard target rates.

A score will be derived in order to make a pass, borderline or fail decision. This score will be derived using implicit criteria together with specified indicators of potentially dangerous practise. It will be retained for the final decision-making and standard-setting process.

Video assessment of work

For this component, one half-day's office work will be videotaped to assess the practitioner's communication skills and the degree of patient involvement during the visit. A rating form will be used to evaluate this component and the score retained for final decision-making.

Self-assessment

A questionnaire is proposed to evaluate the individual's self-assessment skills and the characteristics of the practice. This questionnaire when scored will yield an 'insight quotient'. For example, it may assess the practitioner's self-assessment against a hypothetical standard. This score will also be retained for final decision-making.

Continuing medical education (CME)

The CME component will be a system of credits in five areas. It will include:

  (i) Credentialing from conferences
 (ii) Self-directed CME with and without objectives
(iii) Credits for off-site non-conference learning activities
 (iv) Teaching
  (v) Surveying or credentialing

These five categories of CME credits will yield points which can be converted to a score. This score must meet the standard which is absolute. That is, a minimum score is necessary to achieve recertification on this component independently of the score for the first three components.

The standards

As noted previously, the CME component will have an absolute standard. The college, however, is proposing to evaluate the first three components (see above) by making them into a single global score, using implicit criteria incorporating an absolute standard decided by the college. The decision made on the basis of this global score, would be defended before the recertification board. The final decision would be pass, borderline, or fail with recommendations.

While this process would sample widely, it would be crucial that minimal criteria be established for decision making when possible to minimize bias. The specified structure of the process and sampling would be likely to increase the reliability of the process. Nonetheless, the process is designed to deal with the highly individualistic nature of practice and yet retain enough structure in the evaluation scheme so as to yield as much reliability as possible. The proposal represents a series of trade-offs to make the process as fair and as valid as possible.

Setting standards in maintenance of competence programmes (MOCs): a special problem

Few would be willing to debate the desirability of competence of physicians or the need for their continuing involvement in medical education throughout their professional life. However, many would state that involvement in such programmes alone, without assessment of competence and/or performance, is insufficient for the purpose of recertification.

Whatever the merits of this argument, those organizations which chose the route without an examination component will need to develop standards against which to judge the programme itself and the practitioner's involvement in it. Accumulation of CME credit points as the sole indicator of satisfactory completion of requirements seems to be hardly sufficient!

Standards for MOCs must be based on the principles that underpin adult learning:

(i) The needs of the practitioner should be identified. These needs should reflect more than personal interest: they should be based on structured self-assessment of competence and should include considerations of the physician's profile of practice and the characteristics of the community in which the candidate works

(ii) The education programme should be tailored to meet the identified needs. It should be personalized, multidimensional and should focus on development of skills. Objectives should be defined

(iii) There should be evidence of participation, not just a receipt of registration at a meeting. Ideally, the experience should be interactive and involve the physician in on-going formative assessment

(iv) Evaluation of the appropriateness of the process and its outcome must occur. The 'needs–education–outcome' loop should be closed. Were the physician's learning objectives met? Is the candidate better skilled to handle day-to-day practice? What changes have been introduced as a result of the programme? What new needs have been identified?

As can be seen, more attention needs to be paid to standard setting and monitoring compliance of MOC. Hopefully, innovative approaches will be forthcoming.

Legal issues and consequences

The most obvious consequence of a recertification programme is that some candidates will fail. The approach of the recertification process must be preventive as well as fair. Hence the concept of a 'lead time' is crucial. Candidates and recertifying bodies must design a system that permits early 'testing' leading up to a temporal deadline such that a candidate may or must correct the problem areas by the termination date of the candidate's current certificate.

Recertifying bodies must recognize the fiscal and appointment consequences of failure for practitioners. This may have devastating consequences in certain situations and, without a support structure and fair standards, legal challenges can be expected.

Addition consequences with legal implications will be the status of:

(i) The lifetime certificant

(ii) The foreign-based qualification or so-called equivalency issue as will be seen shortly in the European Economic Community

Most legal challenges will focus around the recertification process and its application to individual candidates. These issues must be anticipated and can often be prevented by observing the following strategies and principles (for a more detailed discussion, see O'Brien (1986), Dauphinee *et al.* (1988), Irby & Milan (1989)):

(i) Documentation is critically important
  (a) Materials clearly defining all steps of the process must be presented in advance of registration for recertification to all candidates
  (b) All decisions on individual candidates must be recorded including the data and facts on which the decision was made. Very importantly, and often neglected, conclusions and global judgements must be based on recorded data
(ii) The content must be fair and therefore job related
(iii) Standard setting must be fair and perceived to be fair. That is to say, it cannot be capricious or arbitrary in reality and in perception
(iv) When soft criteria are applied, the use of multiple judges is recommended
(v) At all times, due process must be observed, including the candidates' right to the last word and appeal before a final decision is made

Summary

As noted in the introduction, all evaluations require a final judgement about the meaning of the data gathered and measurements taken. Does the candidate pass or fail? Standard setting is the process by which one arrives at that final judgement in the most valid and fairest manner. With newer approaches to assessment, new challenges to and applications of standard-setting methods have appeared. In addition, the move towards absolute or criterion-based standards has also had significant impact on the field. These challenges and new approaches apply to standard setting in recertification as much as certification.

With this in mind, the approaches and challenges specific to the emerging field of recertification have been reviewed. Since standard setting for medical practitioners must involve informed professional judgement, it is important that clinicians understand the process and alternatives which measurement experts will present to them. Hence, we have pointed out the general principles as well as issues specific to recertification. Examples have been presented to allow the reader to consider choices in standard setting actively. The objective has been to introduce the reader to the role of a member on a standard-setting committee dealing with recertification. The material may also be of use to members of professional bodies who need a primer on standards as they set out on the road to a recertification process.

References

Angoff, W. F. (1971). Scales, norms and equivalent scores. In *Educational Measurement*, 2nd edn, ed. R. L. Thorndike, pp. 508–600. Washington: Council on Education.

Berk, R. A. (1986). A consumer's guide to setting performance standards on criterion, referenced tests. *Review of Educational Research*, **56**, 137–72.

Dauphinee, W. D., Norman, G., Stillman, P. & Swanson, D. (1988). Residency directors role in assessment of clinical competence. *Annals of the Royal College of Physicians and Surgeons of Canada*, **21**, 35–40.

Ebel, R. C. (1979). *Essentials of Educational Measurement*, 3rd edn. Englewood Cliffs: Prentice Hall.

Hofstee, W. K. B. (1983). The case for compromise in educational testing and grading. In *On Educational Testing*, ed. S. B. Anderson & J. S. Helmick, pp. 109–27. San Francisco: Jossey-Bass.

Holmes, S. E. (1986). Test equating and credentialing examinations. *Evaluation and the Health Professions*, **9**, 230–49.

Irby, D. M. & Milan, S. (1989). The legal context for evaluating and dismissing medical students and residents. *Academic Medicine*, **54**, 639–43.

McLean, L. D., Dauphinee, W. D. & Rothman, A. R. (1988). The oral examination in Internal Medicine. *Annals of the Royal College of Physicians and Surgeons of Canada*, **21**, 510–14.

Nedelsky, L. (1954). Absolute grading standards for objective tests. *Educational and Psychological Measurement*, **14**, 3–19.

Norcini, J. J., Diserens, D. & Day, S. C. *et al.* (1990). The scoring and reproducibility of an essay test of clinical judgement. *Academic Medicine*, **65**, S41–2.

O'Brien, T. L. (1986). Legal trends affecting the validity of credentialing examinations. *Evaluation and the Health Professions*, **9**, 171–85.

Schumacher, C. F. (1978). Reliability, validity and standard setting. In *Measuring Medical Education: the Tests and the Experience of the National Board of Medical Examiners*, 2nd edn, ed. J. P. Hubbard, pp. 59–71. Philadelphia: Lea & Febiger.

16

Implementing a maintenance of competence programme

ROGER GABB (Editor), BRENDAN DOOLEY,
GRAHAME FELETTI, GARRY PHILLIPS,
STEPHEN WEALTHALL and GREGORY
WHELAN

The decision of a college or specialty board to introduce a programme aimed at maintaining the competence of its fellows, members or diplomates is a politically sensitive one. This is particularly true if the maintenance of competence (MOC) programme is associated with recertification. The obvious reason for this is the threat which is inherent in such a system to the status of the current practitioners and, in some cases, to their continuing right to practise in the specialty. For these and other reasons, the debate which leads to the introduction of a MOC programme may be prolonged and sometimes heated. However, the difficulties in introducing a MOC programme do not end with the passing of a series of resolutions which enable the introduction of the programme. The ultimate effectiveness of the programme is likely to depend very much on how the organization goes about the complex business of its implementation. In this chapter some of the issues which deserve consideration in such a situation are explored.

The only assumption made in writing this chapter is that a professional body has resolved to introduce a programme aimed at maintaining the competence of its members. No assumptions are made concerning the methods, content or standards of the programme, nor is it assumed that the programme is a mandatory one linked to recertification or relicensure. It could equally well be a programme based on assessment of competence by formal examination, assessment of performance by practice audit, participation in local quality assurance activities and/or participation in continuing education activities. However, much of the discussion which led to this paper was influenced by the experience of the Royal Australian College of Obstetricians and Gynaecologists in the introduction of its programme of recertification of its Fellows which is

216

based on documented participation in continuing education and quality assurance activities (RACOG, 1989).

Key action areas

The success of the MOC programme will depend very largely on how well the college performs in a number of key areas during the implementation period. While these will vary somewhat depending on the focus of the programme, the following areas deserve attention in most situations.

Survey of members

Collection of information from the membership by means of a survey has proved to be useful in the introduction of a MOC programme in several Australasian colleges (e.g. Hewson, 1989). If it has not been done as part of the development process leading to the policy decision to introduce the MOC programme, it should be done at an early stage in the implementation process. Such a survey serves a number of purposes.

Firstly, it provides data to guide decision-making during implementation. For example, it can be used to collect information on the MOC activities in which members already participate, on the perceived needs of members for MOC activities, on their preferences for various MOC options, and on probable barriers and constraints to participation. Secondly, it can be used to educate the membership about the options which are being considered. While care must be taken to ensure that the educational function of the survey does not distort its data collection function, there is no doubt that such surveys can play a part in sensitizing respondents to some of the issues involved in establishing a MOC programme. Finally, it serves a useful political purpose because it demonstrates to the members that they are being consulted in the development of the programme. This is, of course, effective only if the programme developers respond to the major issues identified in the survey. For example, if the survey shows that there is a large number of members with special needs and these are not catered for in the programme, the survey will have a negative political effect, at least for these members.

The methods used for the survey will, no doubt, reflect the size and geographical distribution of the membership, the resources of the organization and the expertise available. However, the following three-step process is flexible enough to be adapted to most situations. The first step is to interview or to run focus groups with a small sample of members in order to establish what issues are worthy of inclusion in a more extensive study. The participants should include both opinion leaders and representatives of the rank and file membership. The second step is to conduct a more extensive survey of the membership, probably by means of postal questionnaires. The sample selected for this survey will depend on the size and heterogeneity of the membership. In cases where the total membership is relatively small, say less than 2000, it may be sensible to conduct a census of all members. While this may not be required in order to obtain statistically valid results, it may be done in order both to educate and to reassure all members that they are being consulted. The final step may be to interview a sample of members to clarify or to extend issues which were raised in the analysis of questionnaire responses.

Marketing the programme

The next key action is to market the programme. The word 'market' is used here quite deliberately, despite its commercial connotations. The 'product' being marketed in this case is one which is new and threatening to potential 'consumers'. Therefore, the 'marketing campaign' will need both to inform members of the programme and to persuade them that it is in their interests to participate. Viewed from this perspective, one of the key roles of the programme director is that of 'marketing director' and the survey of members can be seen as essential 'market research'. The 'marketing campaign', which should include a 'product launch', needs careful planning. Consideration must be given to both the messages which will be transmitted and the vehicles which will be used to transmit the messages.

Messages

The messages must include both detailed information about the programme which is to be implemented and justification for its introduction. While due consideration must be given to presenting programme details in a way which reduces member anxiety, there is no place for withholding information which is particularly threatening or, indeed, for providing disinformation. Members must be advised honestly of all the features of the programme, including the likely consequences of failing to meet its requirements. At the same time, they must be presented with well-argued rationales for the programme which has been chosen. If the main (or only) purpose of the programme is to encourage continuous improvement and not to identify 'bad apples' (Berwick, 1989; see Chapter 5), this must be made clear early in the marketing campaign. If this is not done, Australian experience suggests that some members will assume that the programme is designed to identify 'bad apples' and will be disappointed when they realize that it cannot perform this function.

Suitable messages which justify the introduction of the programme might include therefore the arguments that: self-regulation is an essential element of professional activity; self-regulation of this type will lead to enhancement of the image of the profession in the eyes of consumers, government and fellow professionals; the introduction of effective self-regulation strategies will protect the professional group from external regulation by government agencies. Sadly, but perhaps inevitably, the defensive argument that 'if we don't do it to ourselves, then someone else will do it to us' seems to be the one which has proved most persuasive to many professionals.

The marketing campaign should also utilize the results of the 'market research' survey. If the programme reflects accurately the preferences of members expressed in the survey, then the argument that a majority of respondents favoured key features of the programme can be used ('You asked for it!'). Alternatively, if the programme planners have introduced features which were not favoured by respondents to the survey, then these differences should not be hidden but addressed explicitly in the campaign ('You didn't ask for this, but you would have if you'd known what we know now!'). Any attempt to 'smuggle' such differences through should be resisted.

Additional messages might stress the established feasibility of the programme, if similar programmes have proved workable in equivalent organizations. Members will also be concerned about the cost of the programme. This concern must also be addressed in the campaign. At the same time, the likely benefits of the programme need to be highlighted so that the marketing message is that the programme, while costly, will provide value for money.

Confidentiality of member records also deserves some emphasis in the campaign. Members must be assured that records of involvement in the MOC programme will be accessible only to the member concerned and to those responsible for administering the programme. However, this assurance may apply only to members in the process of meeting the MOC requirements. When a member fails to meet these requirements, protecting the privacy of the individual member may be seen as less important than protecting both the professional group and the community at large. In this situation, the organization may feel obliged to publish and/or advise regulatory bodies of the names of defaulting members. If so, members need to know this well before the event. Forthright action of this type is likely to be interpreted as a positive aspect of the 'product' by some members, while others will see it as a highly threatening negative aspect.

The most important marketing message is that the programme is 'member friendly' because it is positive (concerned with maintaining high standards of practice) rather than negative (concerned with punishing substandard practice). Many programmes can also be described as 'member friendly' because they are based on existing activities and therefore do not make great demands on most participants in terms of time or money. Finally, the organization must reassure members that it too is 'member friendly' because it will monitor the programme and make modifications if it does not meet the needs of most members. This monitoring can be demonstrated by providing frequent progress reports on the developing programme, including levels of compliance.

Vehicles

All professional bodies will already have some vehicles for communication with their members. These may include printed materials, such as newsletters, bulletins or journals, and face-to-face meetings for both administrative and educational purposes. These existing vehicles should obviously be used in the marketing campaign. The printed publications should include frequent contributions on the programme from the president or chairman as well as from the programme director. At the same time, any meeting attended by significant numbers of members should be used as a forum for advising members of features of the programme and obtaining feedback from members.

More difficult to access, but very important because of their influence, are the informal networks which exist in all organizations. Some consideration needs to be given on how best to use networks such as those which are based on doctors' lounges in hospitals. In some cases it may be necessary to target members who are particularly influential in these networks and to approach them individually in order to gain their support for the programme.

The launch of a new 'product' like a MOC programme to the members of the organization will, however, also require new vehicles dedicated to this purpose. Thus, pamphlets describing the programme may be printed and a newsletter dedicated to the programme may be launched. In addition, consideration should be given to other vehicles, such as video and audio programmes containing presentations by key players, interviews with satisfied members from other bodies which already have a similar MOC programme. A toll-free telephone 'hotline' has also been used successfully by many organizations. Another option which should be considered is a 'travelling circus' in which key players, such as the president or programme director, run a series of consultation meetings around the country. The key to the success of such meetings is to make them opportunities for dialogue rather than one-way lectures. Ideally, some meetings might be held away from major centres so that the concerns of non-metropolitan members can be sought. Alternatively, telephone conferences can be used to encourage the participation of isolated members.

Public relations

As well as marketing the MOC programme to the members of the organization it is also necessary to market it externally. One of the common aims of introducing such a programme is to reassure external agencies that the organization is committed to the maintenance of competence. It cannot be taken for granted that such agencies will learn of the introduction of the programme or that what they learn will be accurate. For this reason, providing clear and precise information on the programme to external agencies must be seen as a key action area which should be addressed early in the implementation period. Groups which may be targeted for this purpose include government agencies, registration/licensure bodies, health insurance organizations (private and public), medical defence insurers, employing agencies (e.g. hospitals), hospital accreditation agencies (e.g. Joint Commission on Accreditation of Healthcare Organizations in the USA, Australian Council for Healthcare Standards in Australia), other professional organizations (e.g. specialty societies or colleges), and consumer groups.

Another reason for ensuring that external agencies are informed of the programme is that some may be involved in actions resulting from non-compliance with the MOC programme. For example, if the programme is a recertification programme, a decision not to recertify a member may have implications regarding the continuing registration/licensure of that member. Similarly, loss of certification may affect the member's status with health insurance organizations or medical defence insurers. Again, it cannot be assumed that these agencies will automatically appreciate the significance of the MOC programme to their concerns, nor can it be assumed that they will act in a way which supports the organization's endeavours. An active programme of information and consultation will be required. In some cases, the proposed MOC programme may need to be modified to meet the needs of key agencies, especially if they are involved in providing the sanctions or 'teeth' of the programme.

Training

Depending on the model of MOC programme chosen, there may be a need for training members in the skills required for its implementation. For example, a MOC programme based on assessment of clinical performance by means of practice audit will demand a substantial number of assessors or auditors (McAuley *et al.*, 1990). The skills required for this task will probably not already exist in the membership and a programme of professional development will be required therefore to train a corps of assessors. Similarly, although it will involve participants other than members, a MOC programme which includes the use of standardized patients in the assessment of competence will demand a substantial training programme before its implementation (Barrows, 1987). If the MOC programme does demand such intensive preparation of members or others, the provision of training programmes must be made a key action area.

Evaluation of the programme

Evaluation must be considered at an early stage and made an integral part of the programme from its inception. This evaluation should be both formative, providing information which can be used to improve the programme, and summative, providing measures of the impact of the programme. Measures of impact can include changes in health care outcomes, member performance, member competence and member participation in MOC activities (Wolf, 1985). In addition, the impact of the programme on other professional activities, such as CME programmes and postgraduate training programmes, can also be studied.

While the importance of evaluation is well recognized, it must be acknowledged that establishing the effectiveness of a national MOC programme is not a job for the faint hearted, since it presents some substantial difficulties. Ideally, what is required for impact evaluation are reliable indicators of the quality of care defined in terms of competence, performance or, preferably, health outcomes. The first difficulty is that widely accepted indicators of overall quality of care just do not exist in most professional areas. The next difficulty is that a randomized controlled trial of such a national programme is not feasible. The best that can be hoped for is the monitoring of these indicators over the period of implementation, a type of quasi-experimental pretest–posttest comparison with the problems of interpretation that are inherent in all uncontrolled studies. In comparison to this type of global programme evaluation, the evaluation of the impact of defined components of the programme will be simpler and, almost certainly, of greater utility in improving the effectiveness of the programme.

Resources

The required resources, both human and material, will depend very much on the type of programme to be implemented. A programme based on peer assessment of clinical performance by means of *in situ* practice audit will clearly demand more resources than one based on multiple-choice question (MCQ) examinations or accumulation of continuing medical education (CME) credits. Nonetheless, there are some common requirements which must be addressed regardless of the type of programme.

Programme director

One of the most critical actions is the appointment of a programme director with responsibility for the implementation of the programme. This is a key political appointment and requires a member who is well known and widely respected by the membership. In making the appointment, consideration needs to be given to the tension which sometimes exists between members in private practice and those in full-time hospital or academic practice. As a MOC system is likely to be seen as more onerous by those in private practice, it may be wise to consider appointing a successful private practitioner as the foundation programme director.
The qualities of the ideal programme director include flexibility and creativity. He or she must be a skilled communicator both in print and in person. The programme director must also be given a high level of autonomy so that he or she can act effectively between the sometimes infrequent meetings of the board or council. The programme director

should also be appointed as chairman of the committee responsible for the programme and should *ex-officio* be a member of the governing body of the organization.

Programme manager

While the programme director plays a critical role in guiding the implementation of the programme, it is difficult to imagine how any but the smallest organizations could mount an effective MOC programme without employing staff members to assist in the development and implementation process. Again, the requirements for staff will depend on the type of MOC programme and the size of the organization, but it seems likely that most will need to appoint at least a full-time programme manager, appropriately supported by administrative staff. The post of programme manager could be filled successfully by a practising member of the organization but it seems likely that many bodies will choose to strengthen their educational expertise by appointing an educationist to this position. Ideally, the programme manager should be a generalist with experience in educational research and development, preferably in medical education, or professional development in another profession. It may also be necessary to employ consultants from time to time to undertake specialized tasks such as surveys, evaluation studies or test development.

Database development

Whatever type of MOC programme is to be implemented, it will almost certainly be necessary to develop a computer database of the MOC activities. This database can be used to generate regular letters advising participants of the MOC activities they have been credited with and of critical dates in a recertification system. It also provides data for regular monitoring of the performance of the programme as part of the ongoing evaluation of the system.

Most MOC programmes require more comprehensive computer support than do certification programmes. There are two main reasons for this. Firstly, the numbers involved are larger, since many MOC programmes involve the entire active membership of the professional group rather than the comparatively small number of candidates engaged at any one time in postgraduate training. Secondly, because MOC programmes cater for members in a wide range of practice situations, they must provide a range of different options to cater for this diversity. This increases the complexity of record keeping and reporting.

Budget

The budget will reflect the model of MOC programme being implemented and the number of participants involved. However, some general considerations apply. It will be necessary to draw up a draft budget at an early stage and this will require determination of how the programme is to be funded. A number of possibilities exist. Firstly, the programme may be funded wholly or in part from general revenue. This will require an increase in subscription dues in most organizations. Secondly, the programme may be funded wholly or in part by an annual MOC levy in addition to the normal annual subscription. The net effect of this option is the same as the first, an increase in annual fees. The only difference is that in the second the moiety dedicated to the MOC programme is identified. Thirdly, the programme may be funded wholly or in part on a 'user pays' basis, with those involved in various activities paying directly for those services. Thus, a programme based on participation in CME activities may be funded from the fees charged for those activities and a recertification programme based on practice audit may be funded from the fees charged to members for auditing their practices. What is perhaps most likely is that some form of mixed funding is chosen with some of the cost being spread across all members and the rest being recovered from those involved in specific activities.

Administrative arrangements

MOC committee

The membership of the committee which is responsible for the programme (which may, for example, be an existing CME or quality assurance committee) must represent the main interest groups within the specialty. It is particularly important that the committee is not dominated by academics and that practitioners are represented adequately. It may be necessary to include representatives of professional subgroups to ensure that the programme meets the needs of the members of these groups as well as those of mainstream members. Because the needs of isolated practitioners are different from those of members in major centres, it is important that the special needs of this group are also considered and a non-metropolitan representative may need to be included in the MOC committee.

The chairman of the MOC committee should be the programme director. He or she should have sufficient delegated responsibility to act for the committee between meetings.

Membership review committee

If the programme is a true recertification programme (based on time-limited certification linked to a required level of performance in the MOC programme), it will be necessary to establish some form of membership review committee. This committee will be responsible for reviewing the cases of those who fail to satisfy the requirements for recertification and then making recommendations to the governing body concerning the membership status of such defaulters. This committee may also be charged with reviewing the cases of those who are threatened with decertification for gross breaches of ethical or technical standards rather than with being denied recertification for failing to meet MOC requirements.

In establishing this committee, it is advisable to determine in detail the procedures which will be used in such a review long before these procedures are needed. In drawing up the procedures, legal advice must be taken to ensure that the principles of natural justice are observed. The defaulting member must be given the right of appeal and appeal mechanisms must be built into the procedures, therefore.

The role of the membership review committee is clearly a sensitive one. Loss of membership may have profound effects on the livelihood of the practitioner, either directly through reduction in payment by insurers or indirectly through loss of appointments or privileges. To ensure fair treatment, the committee should have a different membership from that of the committee responsible for the MOC programme. Once again, however, it is important that the committee be broadly representative of subgroups (geographic, subspecialty, etc.) and that its members enjoy the respect of the professional community.

Other issues

Legal issues

A voluntary MOC programme is not likely to present substantial legal problems but a mandatory MOC programme linked to recertification is likely to be challenged legally. For this reason, legal advice must be sought early in the development process. Potential problems can be reduced by ensuring that all members are advised fully of the requirements of the programme and of the procedures which will be followed in the case of those who do not comply with the requirements of the programme. Similarly, record keeping must be meticulous. Despite all this, the organization introducing mandatory recertification must expect to be sued by disgruntled members and should prepare for this contingency.

Part-time practitioners

One of the most difficult tasks in implementing a MOC programme is to accommodate those who are in part-time practice, often older practitioners who are semi-retired. Such doctors often no longer have teaching hospital appointments and their access to MOC activities is reduced considerably. Their practice may be quite limited both in terms of its clinical range and number of patients. At the same time, their income has decreased and some may find it difficult to afford some MOC activities. An argument may be advanced for dealing leniently with such practitioners in a mandatory MOC programme. Against this, however, is the argument that older practitioners are more likely to provide substandard care than their younger colleagues (McAuley *et al.*, 1990). These members may present organizations with difficulties because they are often loyal members who have served the organization well in the past and the collegiate culture is to honour elder statesmen rather than to make demands of them. Nonetheless, unless organizations wish to award a special type of limited certification to such members, the only logical course would seem to be to demand the same performance in MOC activities of all members, irrespective of the number of hours worked or number of patients seen. Doctors who have declared themselves fully retired from active practice should, of course, be excused from MOC requirements.

Non-member practitioners

An issue which is relevant in Australia and New Zealand, at least, is that of the maintenance of competence of practitioners in the specialty who are not members of the appropriate national college. Naturally enough, practitioners who are required to participate in a MOC programme are annoyed when practitioners with different qualifications, who are not members of the college, can practise alongside them without having to meet those requirements. In some countries, like Australia, where payments under the national health insurance system are linked to acceptable qualifications, it may be possible to ensure that all practitioners are members of the college or, at least, members of an organization which has similar MOC requirements to the college (NSQAC, 1990). In less-regulated systems, however, the task of the college may be the more difficult one of convincing a large number of insurers and providers that members of the college provide better care than nonmembers and therefore should be given preferential treatment.

References

Barrows, H. S. (1987). *Simulated (Standardized) Patients and Other Human Simulations*. Chapel Hill: Health Sciences Consortium.

Berwick, D. M. (1989). Continuous improvement as an ideal in health care. *New England Journal of Medicine*, **320**, 53–6.

Hewson, A. D. (1989). The development of the obligatory education and recertification programme of the Royal Australian College of Obstetricians and Gynaecologists: a practical response to the increasing challenges of a modern society. *Medical Teacher*, **11**, 27–37.

McAuley, R. G., Paul, W. M., Morrison, G. H., Beckett, R. F. & Goldsmith, C. H. (1990). Five-year results of the peer assessment program of the College of Physicians and Surgeons of Ontario. *Canadian Medical Association Journal*, **143**, 1193–9.

NSQAC (National Specialist Qualification Advisory Committee of Australia) (1990). *Lists of Recommended Medical Specialties and Appropriate Qualifications*. Canberra: Australian Government Publishing Service.

RACOG (Royal Australian College of Obstetricians and Gynaecologists) (1989). *RACOG Continuing Education Resource Manual*, Vol. 2. East Melbourne: The Royal Australian College of Obstetricians and Gynaecologists.

Wolf, R. M. (1985). Design problems in evaluation. In *Evaluation of Continuing Education in the Health Professions*, ed. S. Abrahamson, pp. 59–72. Boston: Kluwer Nijhoff.

Part E

Conclusion

17

Requirements for action and research in certification and recertification

BRIAN JOLLY, RICHARD WAKEFORD and
DAVID NEWBLE

Changes in medical education have often been inhibited by calls for 'hard evidence' of their effects and by institutional and professional inertia. The assessment of clinical competence is one of the few areas in educational research in which demonstrable, significant and replicable effects have accrued. In brief, many current assessment practices have detrimental effects on the persons being assessed before, during and after the assessment has taken place. Assessment is often too cursory to make very much sense of the results. Even when designed appropriately, testing methods tend to be concentrated on factual knowledge or basic clinical skills and rarely to address equally important issues like ethics, problem solving or efficiency.

This book has attempted to detail, on an international front, the considerable progress made towards reliable, valid, feasible and sensible assessment of clinical competence. Yet a great deal remains to be done. Inscrutable assessment practices still exist. For example, the importance of detailed feedback to candidates after assessment is ignored persistently and even outlawed by some bodies responsible for assessment, especially at the undergraduate level. Perhaps the most pertinent and unpalatable issue is that, in general, the amount of assessment which takes place is totally inadequate to support the judgements derived from it.

The findings reviewed in the preceding chapters and suggestions offered are, in a few cases, immediately applicable in practice. However, opportunities for action are outnumbered heavily by requirements for more research. In this chapter, we look at several issues on which action might be taken and outline some areas for future study.

Validity

Real life

To achieve valid assessments of clinical competence it is plain that more use will need to be made of 'real life' events and practice. Throughout the book, from the location of assessment 'in training' to the use of practice profiles in determining the content of recertification procedures, justifiable emphasis has been placed on using the real world as the basic building block of assessment technology. The problem is how to do this in a way which yields results which are as rigorous as those provided by more conventional examination methods (multiple-choice questions (MCQs), patient management problems (PMPs), objective structured clinical examinations (OSCEs) and the like). Primarily this must be done by strategically sampling tasks, jobs and roles for collation into tests rather than the other way around. A first approach is to establish the validity of assessments directly by comparing the proposed content with the real events upon which they are based, rather than by using indirect approaches such as correlations between scores on various components of assessment (see Chapter 8). In such an approach, traditional MCQ tests of knowledge would be used rarely, being far removed from real life on the fidelity scale (see Chapter 8). Written tests, including new types of MCQ test, would be based on clinical scenarios and answers would require more discrimination and judgement (Swanson *et al.*, 1991). Simulations would be used more extensively and their validity assessed more rigorously by measuring how outcomes in the simulations compare with outcomes in the real-life situations upon which they were based (Hermann, 1967; Jolly, 1982).

Blueprints

One of the reasons that content validity has been underemphasized so persistently is because in traditional psychological testing content sometimes needs to be concealed from examinees. However, our needs in clinical assessment are quite different. The content should be made quite explicit, since both students and teachers (examiners) need to be quite clear as to what must be achieved if competence is to be certified. It is recommended that a blueprint approach be adopted (see Chapter 6). The content of assessment should be monitored to assure continuing validity while remembering the need for a constant vigil against bias. Even a simple factor like a change of course-team leadership can affect the content validity of course assessment radically.

Involving patients

With the move to evaluating performance in the real clinical setting, patients have the potential to provide much useful data and the only alternative to practice-based peer assessment. Standardized patients have been used successfully in clinical assessments already (Rethans *et al.*, 1991). While this method represents only a small input of the 'patient' or layperson into the assessment process, usually under the controlling influence of the profession, it nevertheless fulfils a useful role. However, the increasing priority given to the rights and preferences of consumers of health services should provide an opportunity to involve more patients in the selection, design and implementation of assessment procedures. This is likely to be particularly appropriate in recertification, which is designed to ensure accountability to the public who are entitled to the highest possible standards of health care (see Chapter 12). This has been reinforced in Chapter 13 where it is suggested that patients should be included in the reference groups who define appropriate domains of interest. In addition, there may be roles, not merely in the delivery of assessment tasks and clinical situations, but also in the establishment of policy and suitable objectives. After all, it was pressure from the public which was partly responsible for the emergence of ethics and communication skills as important goals in undergraduate curricula and the medical profession (Feletti, 1989). The precise way in which patients should be used in assessments must be a matter for further research.

Content specificity

One inescapable fact that has emerged from recent work on the assessment of clinical competence is that inferences ought to be limited to the boundaries of a particular case or patient problem. To obtain a reliable estimate of an examinee's true ability, a large sample of performance on a wide range of cases or problems is required. This finding is not a comfortable one for organizations and examiners dependent for generations on the traditional clinical examination, composed as it is of a very limited sample often restricted to one 'long' case and a few 'short' cases. Moreover, it is somewhat counterintuitive and contradictory to the widely held views about the nature of competence. For example, it is generally believed that doctors can deal with most problems most of the time, while the evidence so far suggests this may be a rash assumption. The concept of general competence is also evident in Chapter 13 of this book.

In Chapter 13 a model of recertification is presented in which a 'common core of practice' is held to have great importance for the way in which the assessments are constructed. This core is seen as 'a set of . . . enduring characteristics of professional medical practice' which contains 'the knowledge, skills and attitudes which all doctors who engage in independent practice in any branch of the profession, including the non-clinical branches, should exhibit'. While it is possible to see the essential characteristics of practice as a cluster of common tasks and responsibilities, it is very difficult to envisage that these, once internalized by clinicians, do not constitute a generic skill or trait. The ability to empathize with and to communicate with patients is an example of such a cluster of skills which seem more like a trait.

Why then are some assessments so context specific? In general, we do not know the answer to this question. It is possible that clinical problem-solving is so dependent on a context-specific knowledge-base that its measurement will remain enigmatic. It is equally possible that some generic traits do exist, but that measurements of them are so contaminated by context-specific attributes as to make them appear less durable than traits should be.

This area requires considerable research, if only because it is highly controversial and, as we have said, counterintuitive. It is important to distinguish between those skills which might be generic and those which are contextual. It is also vital to measure how much an extensive knowledge-base contributes towards apparently contextual skills, mainly for reasons of efficiency of testing. If we wish to construct complex tests of problem-solving ability, which itself is underpinned by a 'conceptually rich and rational knowledge base' (Chapter 8), screening tests tapping that base would obviate the need to give the more complex tests to all candidates. Although some examination boards and colleges appear to use such an approach through the use of qualifying MCQ examinations, the new approach would be radically different. Screening tests would have blueprints, and would be task based and appropriately validated.

National *vs.* local accreditation

Certification procedures vary widely throughout the world. National and local schemes have both advantages and disadvantages. In North America, national schemes predominate. But nationally based assessment schemes should not necessarily be seen as inhibiting experimentation. Paradoxically, in the UK, where certification of undergraduates is still organized at the local (medical school) level, the curricula and examination procedures of the 26 schools show little diversity and certainly do not contain a Harvard, a McMaster or a Beer Sheva. In the UK, the General Medical Council (GMC) has recently issued guidelines encouraging curricular reorganization (GMC, 1991). However, in the past such recommendations have produced little change. It may be that the only way to ensure that these are implemented is through modifying assessment procedures. While instituting a national examination would be a daunting task, some moderating body run on the lines of the UK National Council for Vocational Qualifications may be the only way to get substantial change into both UK curricula and assessment systems. Moves towards some form of national competency-based assessment are also being mooted in Australia.

The main advantage of local examinations is that they can contain a substantial clinical component. The problem in North America is how to implement a clinical component in qualifying examinations which are both psychometrically sound and feasible. This problem also exercises specialty boards and colleges which conduct examinations of competence whose reliability and validity are being challenged.

Effects of assessment on the learning process

One of the major problems, for both locally and nationally organized assessments, is their effect on the participants' learning – mainly in terms of the activities they engage in and the intentions they bring to bear on their study. Wakeford & Southgate (1992) have shown how, in a national examination, introducing a paper designed to test candidates' critical reading skills can increase substantially the amount of attention paid to clinical and research journals. This complements a growing body of knowledge on such effects at the undergraduate level, reviewed in Chapter 8 (see also Jolly *et al.*, 1993). Usually these effects are deleterious, resulting in students cramming knowledge into their short-term memories for regurgitation in factually overburdened examinations. How this effect can be utilized constructively will need considerable thought and research.

Efficiency of assessment

The problem of content specificity discussed in an earlier section has identified the need for a more extensive sampling of students' performance on clinical tasks, irrespective of the test methods being used. The inevitable outcome of this is a requirement for extended testing time with its important resource implications. Limited investigations have been conducted on strategies directed at minimizing this problem (see Chapters 6 and 8). However, both in-training assessment and sequential testing seem essential and some research has begun already (Colliver *et al.*, 1991; Rothman *et al.*, 1992). As far as sequential testing is concerned, issues for research include: the efficiency of various cut-off points; the content and predictive validity of the initial and final parts of the examination; the effect of the initial tests on student learning behaviour; and its acceptability to candidates.

Bias

Bias is commonly thought of as unwanted error in assessment situations, usually where some characteristic not being assessed has an influence on the assessment of the competence of interest (see Chapters 6 and 11). Nevertheless, for most examinations and in-training assessment bias is ubiquitous. It is the main reason for including external moderation in examinations, and for having two examiners at oral/viva voce examinations. However, bias is still poorly understood and researched, probably because more effort has gone into eliminating it (however inadequately) than into measuring it. For example, it is not uncommon for accusations of racial bias to be made against certifying examinations (Anwar, 1987). In some such examinations, effects which might be interpreted as bias have been studied (Jolly *et al.*, 1988; Wakeford *et al.*, 1992). In the former study, the actual biasing factor was non-English mother tongue rather than the racial origin of the candidates. But bias must also be considered in relation to content and predictive validity of examinations. When bias occurs it is often not known precisely what is the real biasing factor (because it has not been measured independently of other variables) and whether the assessment is in fact inadvertently sampling linguistic, social or other factors which are not related directly to the competencies being evaluated. For example, double negatives in the stems of MCQ questions provide enough problems for fluent speakers of a test's language and must add considerable greater difficulties for a candidate of a different mother tongue. In clinical examinations, oral examiners may find it difficult to equate their own standards of practice and care to candidates from different socio-economic or ethnic communities. In such situations, the actual content of the test varies for different sub-groups of candidates (an issue of content validity) and scores on the test may not generalize to real clinical practice of such subgroups (an issue of predictive validity). These features are almost totally unresearched aspects of clinical assessment situations and represent circumstances analogous to studies of bias in selection procedures (e.g. Powis *et al.*, 1992).

Item banking

Item banking has been used extensively for MCQ-type tests. Efforts have been made at local, national and international levels to develop OSCE station banks (Hart, 1990). The technical details of establishing such banks are discussed in Chapter 6. Additional problems will arise as new test formats are introduced and as the focus of test development swings towards the content as the prime concern rather than the method. If sequential testing becomes a major strategy then much more will need to be known about the characteristics of the items/stations (e.g. item/station with total test correlations) particularly when there are batteries of different tests. Vigilant content validation will be essential.

Standard setting

Problems of standard setting will be bound up closely with the use of new test formats and testing strategies (e.g. screening) and with the move towards criterion-referenced examinations. The major issues here are the extent to which all assessment procedures should and do involve a continuum from licensure to certification through to recertification (see Chapter 9). For example, in Chapter 15, Dauphinee and colleagues discuss the commonality of test units and the possible equation of standards between an MCQ used for certification and a similar test used for recertification. Unless there are means and mechanisms for monitoring the testing policies and practices of various bodies and agencies throughout the continuum of qualification, and unless these strategies become much more professionally scrutable and debatable, appropriate standard setting and scoring will be impossible.

Modifying assessment procedures

Coordinating change

Earlier in this chapter, the lack of change in assessment procedures over the last few years was discussed. Apart from the sheer difficulty of tackling these problems there are several other reasons for this inertia. The recognition that there is a problem has not always been forth-coming. Coordination between undergraduate, postgraduate and health service delivery sectors and institutions has been difficult and in many countries is becoming more so. Often, within any one country, innovative changes have been contained within a few individual institutions, even though they may have reverberated widely abroad (e.g. the OSCE and standardized patients). In the main this has been due to inadequate dissemination, passive conservatism, or the active, but misplaced, belief that current assessment systems were more than adequate. The most pressing need is for those responsible for assessment in medical schools, and professional and government institutions, to become aware of the limitations of the current technology and the advantages of the emerging ones.

If change is to take place a strategy needs to be developed which will encompass several core activities (e.g. maintenance of competence programme, see Chapter 16; Gale & Grant, 1990). The first three of these will involve:

  (i) Establishing the need for change

 (ii) Galvanizing the power to act

(iii) Designing, disseminating and modifying the change itself

We see this book as encompassing the first of these ventures. The second will involve a number of consultative and training initiatives, some of which have already started. For example, a working party of the Austra-lian Medical Council has already been set up to respond to initiatives on competency-based assessment; the Royal College of General Practi-tioners in the UK possesses a forum on assessment; and the specialty boards in the USA have taken important policy decisions on recertification.

Selection and training of examiners

These are issues that have received little attention. Rarely are examiners selected on the basis of any objective measure of their ability to be fair and consistent. Fortunately, recent research shows that examiners contribute less error to an assessment than do other sources (cases, occasions, test methods, etc.) (Swanson & Norcini, 1989) despite the fact that some examiners continue to give inconsistent ratings (Newble *et al.*, 1980; van der Vleuten *et al.*, 1989; Tamblyn *et al.*, 1991). The characteristics and craft knowledge of 'good' versus 'poor' examiners should be investigated thoroughly. It should also be recognized that most of the recent work on the unreliability of assessment has been undertaken in a few institutions in which great lengths are taken to reduce inter-examiner variability by extensive training and calibration. The vast majority of examiners at various levels of medical education receive no formal training or calibration whatsoever. This will be a particular problem if and when in-training assessment (ITA) is implemented. Fair and effective assessment 'at the coal face' will entail a different set of skills and training programmes from the 'big bang' one-off assessment procedures.

Staff development

In Chapters 3 and 4, the importance of building strong staff development programmes for examiners and assessment technicians was highlighted. Indeed it is unlikely that major changes can be accomplished without such efforts. The success of new forms of assessment in the USA and Canada, and the relative lack of resistance to the changes, have probably come about as a result of the comprehensiveness of built-in design and validation exercises for all potential examiners. In this way ownership of the examination and of newer developments has proceeded unobstructed by reactionary influences. The other important feature has been the existence of a small but influential group of clinically qualified and psychometrically competent examination designers, underpinned by extensive technical support. Similar conditions need to prevail in individual medical schools in the USA, UK and Australia, and at national accrediting institutions in the UK and Australia, if assessment is to become a respectable and valued tool internationally. Workshops, largely staffed by the authors of this book, have been mounted recently. But a much more formal international exchange and development programme in assessment should be constructed.

Modifying candidates' understanding and use of assessment data

An implication of changes in assessment practices and in the use of assessment by examiners is that candidates, especially in ITA (see Chapter 11), need also to change their attitudes towards assessment. Knowledge about the error associated with assessment practices should be available to candidates and consumers of the output of examinations alike. The validation of content (Chapters 6, 7 and 13) should allow much more precise feedback to candidates about their performance, and profiling of their strengths and weaknesses should be possible. This is likely to be resisted strongly, especially by those responsible for certification examinations.

Cost and efficiency

The major implications of more precise assessment are increasing amounts of assessment and rising costs. This is particularly true if 'real life' assessment is to be undertaken. In some cases this means that a bigger proportion of revenue from professional examinations will need to be devoted to the development and maintenance of testing procedures. However, for individual schools which wish to assess validly and reliably, and which do not have open-ended resources, this means considerable extra expenditure. It is in this area where national coordination might be desirable along the lines of the National Board of Medical Examiners in the USA. In the wake of increased patient potency, governments may be persuaded to devote more resources to this field.

Furthermore, rigorous research should be directed towards establishing the validity of time-limited recertification or the value of eligibility criteria in recertification procedures. It is pointless devoting energy to establishing strong assessment systems if they are used at inappropriate times or on the wrong people. Questions need to be answered about the relationship between time and efficiency of 'bad apple' screening, and more details are needed about characteristics of practitioners 'at risk'. The common rules of '5 years' or 'all single-handed practitioners' need empirical support. These studies should go hand in hand with developments and lead to fine tuning at a later stage.

Frontiers

Cognitive psychology

New understandings of the nature of problem-solving and the effects of assessment on student learning and test-taking behaviour is regarded as one of the cutting edges of test development (see Chapter 8). These new concepts will have important implications for the measurement of competence with new methods and approaches already being given trials.

In-training assessment

The introduction of ITA should be seen as an essential part of an effective clinical assessment or maintenance of competence strategy (see Chapters 11 and 16). The major issues here are not methodological. The profession is so wedded to the idea of summative, one-off or hurdle-type assessments that a major reorientation will need to take place before a change towards ITA is possible. For this reason, research and development should be devoted to investigating how the climate of opinion can be modified. An urgent need in relation to MOC is to coordinate the efforts of course designers, teachers, examining bodies and governmental organizations within any one strand of the profession. In this respect Chapter 16 provides the first steps to establishing such a programme. These include: emphasizing the collection of members views; establishing need and feasibility; marketing and public relations; and the development of legal protection and budgeting.

Coordination of assessment and continuing medical education

Chapter 12 focused on the perennial dilemma of the goal of recertification; is it aimed at identifying 'bad apples' or at 'enhancement of competence' (Berwick, 1989)? The answer will determine the focus of continuing medical education (CME), namely rehabilitation or professional development respectively. Either answer may be appropriate in certain circumstances. Whichever predominates will require a separate set of research questions to be answered.

The 'bad apples' approach will require research of a much more detailed and probing nature on the characteristics which predispose towards risk of malfunctioning or low levels of competence. In addition, outcome analysis of retraining programmes and detailed research on practitioners disbarred for other reasons of negligence or ethical transgressions will be required. Searching for 'bad apples' implies that rehabilitation is both desirable and effective.

The 'enhancement of competence' approach entails research of a totally different kind. What is needed is an evaluation of a strategy for running CME programmes which can address the following issues:

(i) What are the needs of practitioners as seen from their own and outside perspectives?

(ii) Do current CME activities meet those needs?

(iii) What CME activities (or financial incentives or legal changes) are perceived as being most beneficial in enhancing practice behaviour?

(iv) How can the providers of CME activities be encouraged to develop training which will strengthen self-assessment and self-directed learning rather than passive reception of new techniques or new knowledge?

(v) By what assessment-related criteria should CME activities be judged? For example, do participants in CME actually organize their practices better, solve problems quicker, become more cost conscious than non-participants? In other words, does the 'enhancement of competence' model actually work?

References

Anwar, M. (1987). *Overseas Doctors: Experience and Expectations.* London: Commission for Racial Equality.

Berwick, D. M. (1989). Continuous improvement as an ideal in health care. *New England Journal of Medicine*, **320**, 53–6.

Colliver, J. A., Mast, T. A., Vu, N. V. & Barrows, H. S. (1991). Sequential testing with a performance based examination using standardised patients. *Academic Medicine*, **66**, S64–S66.

Feletti, G. (1989). 'The patient's view'. In *Views of the Learner: Implications for Assessment*, ed. B. C. Jolly. Paper from the Fourth Cambridge Conference on Medical Education. Cambridge, 5–11 June, 1989.

Gale, R. & Grant, J. (1990). *Managing Change in a Medical Context: Guidelines for Action.* London: British Postgraduate Medical Federation.

GMC (General Medical Council) (1991). *The Future of Undergraduate Medical Education: The Need for Change.* London: General Medical Council.

Hart, I. R. (1990). The OSCE data bank. In *Teaching and Assessing Clinical Competence*, ed. W. Bender, R. J. Hiemstra, A. J. J. A. Scherpbier, R. P. Zwierstra, pp. 28–30. Groningen: BoekWerk Publications.

Hermann, C. F. (1967). Validation problems in games and simulations with special reference to models of international politics. *Behavioural Science*, **12**, 216–31.

Jolly, B. C. (1982). A review of issues in live patient simulation. *Programmed Learning and Educational Technology*, **19**, 99–107.

Jolly, B. C., Cohen, R., Rothman, A. I. & Ross, J. (1988). Graduates of foreign medical schools: demographic and personal predictors of success on an OSCE-format internship programme entrance examination. In *Proceedings of the 27th Annual Conference on Research in Medical Education*, pp. 234–9. Washington: Association of American Medical Colleges, 11–17 November 1988.

Jolly, B. C., Newble, D. I. & Chinner, T. (1993). The learning effect of re-using stations in an Objective Structural Clinical Examination. *Teaching and Learning in Medicine*, **5**, 66–71.

Newble, D. I., Hoare, J. & Sheldrake, P. F. (1980). The selection and training of examiners for clinical examinations. *Medical Education*, **14**, 345–9.

Powis, D., McManus, I. C. & Cleave-Hogg, D. (1992). Selection of medical students: philosophic, political, social and educational bases. *Teaching and Learning in Medicine*, **4**, 25–34.

Rethans, J. J., Sturmans, F., Drop, R. & van der Vleuten, C. (1991). Assessment of performance of general practitioners by the use of standardised (simulated) patients. *British Medical Journal*, **41**, 97–9.

Rothman, A. I., Ross, J., Cohen, R. & Poldre, P. (1992). 'Sequential testing in clinical skills assessment'. Paper presented at the Fifth Ottawa International Conference on the Assessment of Clinical Competence, Dundee.

Swanson, D. & Norcini, J. (1989). Factors influencing the reproducibility of tests using standardised patients. *Teaching and Learning in Medicine*, **1**, 85–91.

Swanson, D., Case, S. & van der Vleuten, C. (1991). Strategies for student assessment. In *The Challenge of Problem Based Learning*, ed. D. Boud & G. Feletti, pp. 260–73. London: Kogan Page.

Tamblyn, R. M., Klass, D. J., Schnabl, G. K. & Kopelow, M. L. (1991). Sources of unreliability and bias in standardized-patient rating. *Teaching and Learning in Medicine*, **3**, 74–85.

van der Vleuten, C. P. M., van Luyk, S. J., van Ballegooijen, A. M. J. & Swanson, D. B. (1989). Training and experience of examiners. *Medical Education*, **23**, 290–6.

Wakeford, R. E. & Southgate, L. (1992). Postgraduate medical education: modifying trainees study approaches by changing the examination. *Teaching and Learning in Medicine*, **4**, 210–13.

Wakeford, R. E., Farooqi, A., Rashid, A. & Southgate, L. (1992). Does the MRCGP examination discriminate against Asian doctors? *British Medical Journal*, **305**, 92–4.

Index